This book is dedicated to Ben, Josh, Katriel, Ellen, and Kayla. You are all my children, whether through birth or marriage. I thank God for each of you every day.

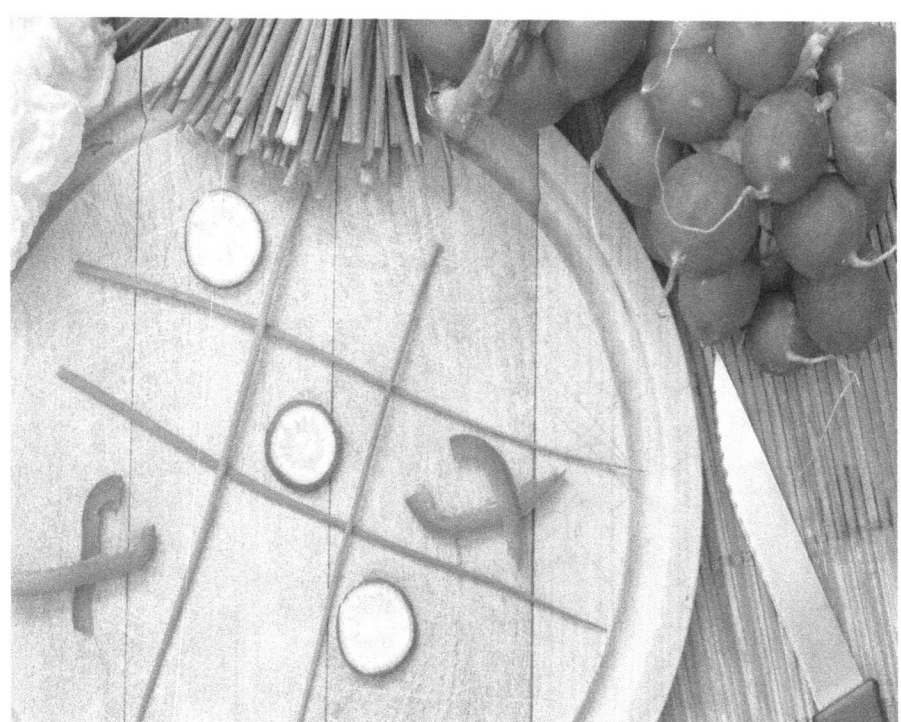

ISBN 10: 1483981118

ISBN 13: 978-1483981116

Other books by Dr. Leanna Manuel

Tap It Away: 10 Minutes to Freedom With EFT

Copyright 2011

ISBN 10: 1477558195

ISBN 13: 978-1477558195

Don't Diet

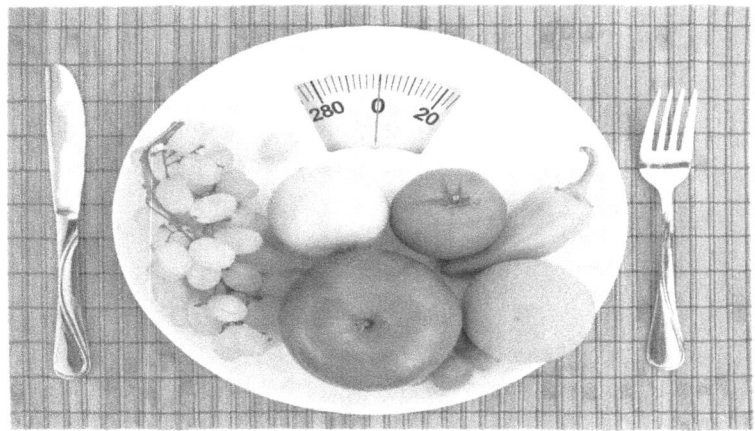

Reprogram Your Weight
With Meridian Tapping

by Dr. Leanna Manuel

Introduction

Every day we are bombarded by media that reinforce the idea that we are not skinny enough, healthy enough, or fit enough. Generally speaking there is substantial evidence for at least two of those. A recent search at www.amazon.com revealed that there have been 5,008 new releases in the last 30 days in the area of Health, Fitness, and Dieting. There have been 16,853 new releases in the last 90 days. A more specific search on the same site indicated 38,606 titles for Diet and Weight Loss and 36,702 releases for Exercise and Fitness. A search of the keyword diet at www.barnesandnoble.com revealed 105,744 titles and a search for weight loss turned up 10,844 titles.

Weight loss programs are available in many different formats including online programs, storefront operations, meeting-based programs, hospital-based programs, residential treatment centers, and boot camps. You can have your meals shipped to your home, drink your meals, count calories, tally up your points, or have surgery. Equally prevalent are the numerous exercise programs that promise revolutionary results. You can go to the gym, work out with a personal trainer, sweat to a DVD, or go to a fitness camp. Whether you look at the weight loss or the exercise options it would appear that there are already plenty of books and programs. With all of the information out there, why do I (and millions of other people) struggle with food and weight?

Most of the exercise programs and diet programs I have ever tried have been good at telling me how to do something. I am well-versed in nutrition, calories, dietary modification, and exercise techniques. I know that you are too. One of the things that has been missing for me in the past is the understanding of WHY I eat. I consume food for a variety of reasons, and hunger is rarely one of them. I eat in response to emotions. I eat in response to habit and schedules. I eat to try to attain a specific mood state. I eat because of imbalances that create cravings. I eat because of disruptions in my body's energy system.

A physician once said to me, "It's simple. Eat less. Exercise more." I knew at that moment that this person didn't know me at all. Nothing could be farther from the truth for me. If it were that simple I would have already done it. I bet you would have too. Was he right that eating less is part of the equation? Sure. But it is only a partial truth. Was he also correct that exercising more is important? Absolutely. What I now know is that unless my body's energy system is in balance, I am completely unable to sustain either of those edicts. The disruptions that are driving my unhealthy relationship with food must be addressed if I am to have any chance for lasting success.

Unlike most of the diet and exercise books I have viewed over my lifetime, this book will not endorse any specific diet. There are no foods to avoid. There is no magic exercise program. This book focuses on WHY we eat and neutralizing the unhealthy relationship we have had with food. There are exercises to help you get more in touch with your own thoughts, feelings and attitudes about food, diet, exercise, and your body. You will also become more aware of how stress, anxiety, anger, and frustration impact your weight, both directly and indirectly.

How to get the most out of this book

To get the most out of this book, start at the beginning and work your way through the first section, one topic at a time. You will learn the basics of meridian tapping including the tapping points, how to use words and phrases to help with focus and energy, and explore the factors that contribute to your own weight loss issues. You will also learn about Psychological Reversal, a significant issue related to the failure of many weight loss and fitness programs.

The second part of the book is a collection of meridian tapping sequences that are specific to exercise, stress eating, body image, cravings, mood, health and medical problems, exercise avoidance, holidays and special occasions, and many other concerns that can sabotage our best-laid plans. As you work through these exercises you are likely to have additional thoughts about the tapping phrases or related experiences. I recommend that you write them down and I will remind you to do this periodically. These journal entries will be the jumping of points for more tapping to enhance your life and health.

Within the tapping section of the book you will find several icons, that should be self-explanatory once you learn the basics of tapping. Don't worry if you don't completely understand right now. The stop sign is a reminder to stop tapping and it will be followed by a reminder to rate the intensity of the feeling on a 0-10 scale.

 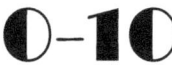 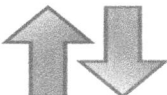

There will then be either a set of arrows like is shown above, or there will be a hand holding a pencil, as shown below. When you see the arrows, this is to suggest returning to the previous tapping if you are still experiencing distress or to continue with the tapping that follows if you are making good progress. When you see the pencil, that is a reminder that writing down your thoughts and feelings is suggested.

 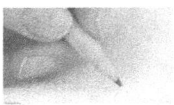

Basic Rationale

You are energy. I am energy. Anything that changes our energy changes our experience of life. That includes our thoughts, our feelings, and our body. The Chinese used this knowledge when they devised the system of acupuncture that manipulates the body's energy to create and maintain health. Through the combined brilliance of several pioneers and methodologies, we have learned how to change our energy in much the same way - but without the needles. Instead of someone sticking you with needles, you are going to gently tap on some of the spots where an acupuncturist would insert needles. Because of this, some people call meridian tapping a form of psychological acupuncture.

We are all energy and we have an energy frequency. Our bodies, our thoughts, and even our feelings are a constantly changing form of electrical energy. The exciting news is that this electrical energy can be changed. I would bet that you have seen images on television or in the movies where there is a flat line on the heart monitor, but then the doctor applies electricity to the person's chest and the heart rate returns. Meridian tapping works in much the same way. A subtle change in the electrical energy applied in one place impacts the electrical energy of your entire system.

Through acupuncture, acupressure, or meridian tapping we can exert influence on the energy system. This influence can change our thoughts, feelings, and even the way our bodies function.

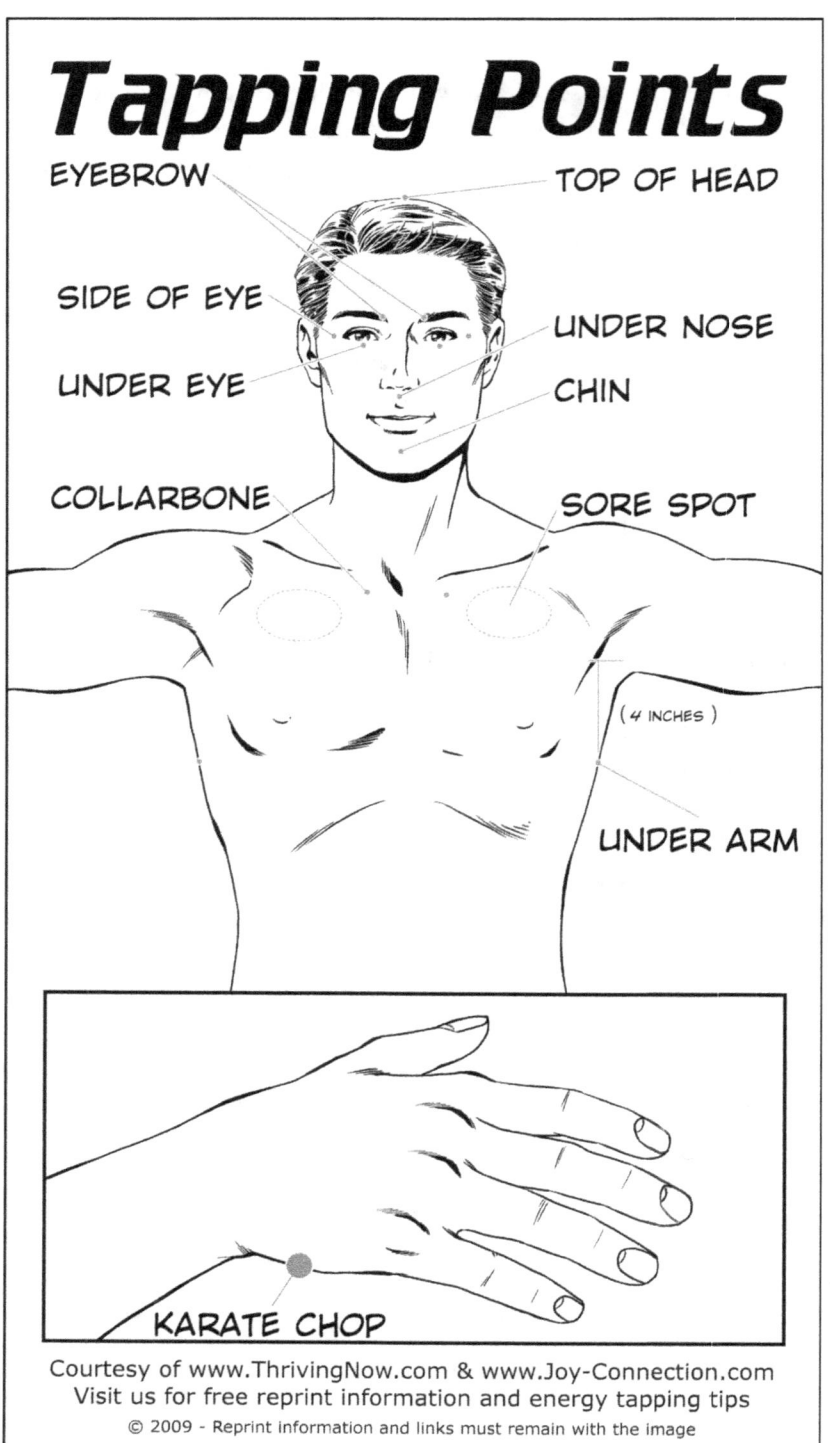

Tapping Points

EYEBROW

TOP OF HEAD

SIDE OF EYE

UNDER NOSE

UNDER EYE

CHIN

COLLARBONE

SORE SPOT

(4 INCHES)

UNDER ARM

KARATE CHOP

Courtesy of www.ThrivingNow.com & www.Joy-Connection.com
Visit us for free reprint information and energy tapping tips
© 2009 - Reprint information and links must remain with the image

Basic Tapping

There are hundreds of acupuncture points on the body. For basic meridian tapping we are only going to use a few of them.

Eyebrow - at the starting point of the eyebrow, beside the bridge of the nose

Side of Eye - at the side of the eye, near the temple

Under the Eye - under the eye, on the orbital bone

Under the Nose -under the middle of the nose

Chin - in the crease between your lower lip and above your chin

Collarbone - just under the collarbone, near the sternum

Under the Arm - about 4 inches below the armpit

Top of Head - on the crown of the head

Karate Chop - on the side of the hand between the little finger and the wrist

These tapping points are generally sufficient to address most people's issues. When you tap on these spots you will tap gently on the area with your fingertips for approximately 7 taps. A diagram of the tapping spots is included for you on the previous page.

Generally, meridian tapping involves 6 steps.

1. Make a statement that describes what needs to change

2. Rate the emotional intensity associated with that statement

3. Repeat a setup statement or statements

4. Tap on the meridians using the tapping points

5. Repeat the original statement

6. Rate the intensity again

Let's practice. Tap 5-9 times on each of the tapping points. Nothing bad will happen if you tap fewer or more times. You don't have to tap hard. Tap firmly enough to feel it, but it shouldn't cause any pain or discomfort.

Meridian Tapping Basics

Tapping Spots

These tapping points have been borrowed from Chinese medicine, specifically acupuncture. I am incredibly relieved that I do not have to understand the how or why of these acupuncture points in order to do meridian tapping. There are so many different acupuncture points on the human body that it is absolutely amazing. I like to think of all of these points as little electrical outlets where I can plug in. The points are very easily recognized and they respond well to external tapping rather than using a needle. I have had acupuncture and have found it to be quite effective and not at all painful, but it just isn't very portable. I can tap on my tapping spots anytime and anywhere, and that makes it so much more convenient for many things.

The basic meridian tapping spots are spread out on some major energy circuits of the body. In Chinese medicine these energy circuits have names that sometimes correspond to body organs, but it is not necessary to get much more into that unless you are interested in actually studying the Chinese medicine philosophies. Each of these energy circuits are then associated with different personality characteristics, disease processes, and symptoms. For our purposes, we really only need to know where they are located. The chart that follows summarizes the most commonly used tapping points, and lists their normal abbreviation, name, and location. Some acupuncture nomenclature is included as well.

EB	Eyebrow	Where eyebrow meets bridge of nose	Bladder2 Meridian
SE	Side of Eye	At the outer corner of the eye, near the temple	Gall Bladder 1 Meridian
UE	Under the Eye	Beneath the eye, in the midline at the top of the cheek	Stomach 2 Meridian
UN	Under the Nose	In the midline, under the nose and above the lip	Governing Vessel 25-26 Meridians

CH	Chin	In the crease below the lip and above the chin	Conception Vessel 24 Meridian
UA	Under Arm	Approximately in line with the male nipple (for women, where the bra rides under the arm)	Spleen 21 Meridian
CB	Collarbone	Directly to the left or right of the sternum in the soft spot just below the collarbone	Kidney 27 Meridian
TH	Top of Head	At the crown of the head	Governing Vessel
KC	Karate Chop	On the outside of the hand, between the base of the pinky and the wrist	Small Intestine 3-4 Meridians

Setup Phrases

Setup phrases can be a very useful prelude to meridian tapping. The setup phrase is the preparation for tapping. It includes a statement of the problem as well as a positive affirmation. There are many ways to construct a setup statement. It can be a simple statement such as "I am hungry" or something much more complex such as a rambling exploration of a problem that is not yet clearly defined in your mind. You will find examples of both types of setup phrases in the tapping exercises that follow. The affirmation is what helps to prepare the body's energy system for change. A traditional affirmation is "I deeply and completely love and accept myself." Even though it is simple, it really works. Other people find that expanding the affirmation feels more useful. This might include a choice statement that outlines what the desired resolution to the problem might be.

Reminder Phrases

Reminder phrases are usually a shortened version of the problem statement that serves to keep us focused on the problem. People have very strong defense mechanisms that are useful to help us avoid the pain of our own circumstances. Although we say that we want to resolve our problems, our natural tendency is to avoid or distract ourselves from the associated pain or discomfort. The reminder phrase prevents our minds from wandering away from the issue. If you use our previous problem statement of "I am hungry" we can use a reminder phrase of "this hunger" to keep us focused.

Basic Negative Sequence

When I first learned meridian tapping it was in the form of EFT - The Emotional Freedom Technique, as taught by Gary Craig. The setup statements and tapping sequences follow a very basic format. The setup phrases, a basic statement of the problem is repeated three times while you tap on the karate chop point. This is followed by "I deeply and completely love and accept myself." The reminder phrase was a shortened version of the problem statement and was repeated at each of the tapping points. This repetitive sequence of setup phrase and reminder phrases was repeated until the intensity rating was significantly reduced. This continues to be the basis of EFT and works remarkably well. It takes very little thought or effort to figure out how to proceed. A thought or feeling comes into your awareness and you can plug it into this simple formula.

> Even though (insert thought or feeling here) I deeply and completely love and accept myself.

Then you can say the thought or feeling as you tap on each of the other tapping points. Or, if it is a long thought or feeling, you can shorten it to just a few key words that will keep you focused on the problem at hand.

These setup statements and reminder phrases are negative statements. They are not intended to be positive. The negative statements and phrases act as the keys to unlock the negative energy that is trapped in our energy system and can play an important part in reclaiming our emotional freedom, resolving problems, and enhancing our wellbeing.

Positive Tapping

EFT purists say it isn't necessary, but many variations of EFT that include additional positive affirmations are wildly popular. I have found that the perfect time to add some positive affirmations while tapping is after you have tapped on the negative statements for a while and your intensity has lowered considerably. I personally do not recommend positive tapping until your negative intensity rating is a 3 or lower.

Most issues resolve with the standard negative sequence. Whether by personal preference or necessity, positive phrases can also be beneficial. Looking back at the earlier problem statement of "I am hungry," we could substitute "I choose to follow my eating plan with confidence" instead of "I deeply and completely love and accept myself." This type of choice statement, made popular by Dr. Patricia Carrington (Carrington, 2001), is very empowering. It extends to the reminder phrases as well. Some of the negative reminder phrases can be replaced with the new resolution or choice statement.

Narrative Technique

An alternative to the repetitive negative or positive phrase technqiues is a narrative technique option. The setup phrase can include various statements and tell a story about the problem or, in a sense, talk to yourself, during the tapping sequence. These statements may continue in the traditional negative format or can take us progressively from a negative state of mind to a more positive state.

Intensity Ratings

I first became aware of rating scales when I was working as a nurse. It was quite common to ask someone to rate their pain. Sometimes we used a 5 point scale, sometimes a 10 point scale, but the purpose was always the same. We were trying to get a way to measure someone's experience at a distinct point in time. Not only was that useful in determining interventions, but it was also valuable in judging the effectiveness of treatments. Also, during my clinical psychology training we frequently constructed and used rating scales. Rating scales are frequently used for the rating of emotions, just as they were for the rating of physical symptoms in my nursing experiences.

The process of rating the intensity of the feeling when engaged in meridian tapping is not essential but can be very useful. As noted above, it can give you a snapshot of your current experience. It becomes particularly beneficial when the feeling changes. Instead of noticing our relief, most of us move very quickly on to the next problem or an aspect of the original problem that we were not previously working on. Then, instead of noticing how well meridian tapping worked to help us and how much better we actually feel, we mistakenly believe that nothing has happened and might even give up on using the technique.

Sometimes, when our intensity about a topic drops dramatically, we feel so much better that we do not finish the process. It is a tremendous relief to go from an intensity level of 10 where you can feel the distress in your whole body down to a level of 5 or 6. If you stop there, you will continue to feel better, but not as good as if you make the issue go away completely. The ratings can be useful to help you stay in touch with what you are really feeling.

The rating scale that I use is identified by the acronym SUDs. It stands for Subjective Units of Distress scale. This scale is defined by the user. When I label my feeling as a 10 it will not be exactly the same as what you rate as a 10. If you are asked to rate the intensity of a bad feeling, with 10 being the worst, it is generally useful to give your first impression and not overthink it too much. Sometimes it can also be helpful to flip the scale around, particularly when tapping on something that you want to increase. I find it helpful to think of 10 being the most of something (good or bad) and 0 being the least (good or bad). For visual people, it can be helpful to see the scale more like a thermometer. You can take a visual reading of your intensity thermometer. Again, low intensity would probably be visualized as a low temperature and high intensity would be visualized as a high temperature.

Unfortunately, many people get hung up on the SUDs rating. They may have difficulty assigning a value and worry about what will happen if they use the wrong number. There is no such thing as the wrong number. As mentioned previously, the amount of feeling, intensity, or distress that you feel is subjective. It is relevant only to you and depends on many factors including your previous experiences, tolerance to pain and discomfort, and the context of your current experience.

Before I had experienced childbirth or knee surgery I might have assigned an intensity level of 10 to a physical pain, believing that it is the worst pain anyone could ever experience. My experience of that pain was real. Then came knee surgery. Retrospectively, the previous physical pain would have only been a 6. Knee surgery pain became my new gold standard for pain intensity. I hope that I never experience anything worse that makes me re-evaluate whether knee surgery was a 10 or not, but who knows? The same is true for emotional states. It can be difficult to rate sadness. People who experience the grief of losing a beloved pet really are sad. They may experience it as a 9 or 10 at the time, but can acknowledge that in comparison to the sadness of losing a child or mate it might be somewhat lower.

The exact number doesn't matter. It isn't to be judged by anyone. It is your own subjective experience which cannot be wrong. Don't let the intensity rating derail you. I do have a tapping exercise for you that may help with any confusion or difficulty you are having. If you are still having difficulty with the ratings after you have tapped - skip them. After you have more experience with tapping you can go back and try the ratings again. It is much more important to do the tapping than to worry about the ratings.

Say this problem statement aloud, "I can't rate the intensity." Is this a little true, or a lot true for you? Guess at the 0-10 number and write it down. Repeat this setup statement three times while tapping on the karate chop point. "Even though I can't seem to rate the intensity of my feeling or experience, I deeply and completely love and accept myself." Now, tap on each of the eight tapping points using a reminder phrase.

Eyebrow	Can't rate the intensity
Side of Eye	Problem with ratings
Under the Eye	Not sure about the intensity
Under the Nose	Anxious about assigning a number
Chin	It might not be right
Collarbone	Afraid to rate the intensity
Under the Arm	Can't rate the intensity
Top of Head	Problems with ratings

Barriers to Getting Started

Apathy and inertia are both factors that can make it difficult to start anything including healthy eating or weight management. Apathy can include the lack of desire, will, or energy to do anything (Kowalick, 1998). In that sense, apathy is a block for starting. Inertia is another block. For most of us, it is difficult to get started from a standstill. This is a very common problem for individuals trying to start an exercise program. Fortunately meridian tapping is a fantastic tool for overcoming these barriers to getting started.

Say this problem statement aloud. "I am stuck." Rate the intensity on the scale of 0-10. Record your rating. Repeat this setup statement three times while gently tapping on the karate chop point. "Even though I feel stuck, I deeply and completely love and accept myself." Now, at each of the eight tapping points, repeat this reminder phrase.

Eyebrow	I am stuck
Side of Eye	I am stuck
Under the Eye	I am stuck
Nose	I am stuck
Chin	I am stuck
Collarbone	I am stuck
Under the Arm	I am stuck
Top of Head	I am stuck

Take a deep breath and check the intensity of your original problem statement. "I am stuck." Repeat this sequence until you no longer feel stuck.

Many people complain that they are not motivated to do things. Only some of the activities we engage in are intrinsically motivating. These are things like eating a hot fudge sundae, soaking in a hot tub, or enjoying a good massage. Most other things are motivating only because they bring something else that is pleasurable into our lives or help us to avoid something unpleasant. Most people who come into my office say they want to be more motivated for all of the activities of life.

Say this problem statement aloud, "I lack motivation." Rate the intensity on the 0-10 scale and record it. Repeat this setup statement three times while tapping on the karate chop point. "Even though I lack motivation and can't seem to find what really does motivate me, I choose to be joyfully surprised by how easy and comfortable it is to enter into a state of flow, where everything happens naturally." At each of the eight tapping points use a different reminder phrase while tapping.

Eyebrow	I am totally unmotivated right now
Side of Eye	I don't feel energized
Under the Eye	Nothing is moving me in any one direction
Under the Nose	Nothing on the outside is motivating me
Chin	Nothing on the inside is motivating me

Collarbone	Incentives and rewards aren't working
Under the Arm	Even punishments aren't working
Top of Head	I am just plain unmotivated

Take a deep breath and check the intensity of your original problem statement. "I lack motivation." Record your rating. Notice whether it is going down or up. If it is going up, consider adding a word or phrase that describes what you are unmotivated to do in the setup and in the sequence, like "I lack motivation to go to the gym."

Continue tapping with these or other similar reminder phrases until your intensity rating is down to a low level. Then, at each of the eight tapping points, use a different reminder phrase while tapping gently.

Eyebrow	I am unmotivated right now
Side of Eye	And I choose to move toward a state of flow anyway
Under the Eye	I don't feel energized right now
Under the Nose	And I choose to set clear goals anyway
Chin	I can't find anything that motivates me right now
Collarbone	And I choose to feel amazingly calm and confident about moving forward anyway
Under the Arm	Nothing has worked so far to get me motivted
Top of Head	And I continue to feel empowered
Eyebrow	I am immune to incentives, rewards, and punishments
Side of Eye	I choose to feel fully involved in my life anyway
Under the Eye	I have been unmotivated
Under the Nose	I choose to remain open to the possibility that things could change
Chin	I don't know what really motivates me

Collarbone	I choose to allow that knowledge into my consciousness
Under the Arm	Motivation is only one way to get moving
Top of Head	I choose to move forward with or without motivtion

Take a deep breath and check the intensity of your original problem statement. "I lack motivation." Record your rating. Repeat the exercise until you can say "I lack motivation" without any real intensity. In other words, repeat the exercise until the statement no longer feels true.

Apathy is different from being unmotivated. When someone is unmotivated they are not necessarily indifferent to the outcome. They only lack the energy or drive to overcome inertia. Apathy can be very destructive and derail us completely from our goals.

Say this problem statement aloud. "I feel apathetic." Rate the intensity you experience when saying this on the 0-10 point scale and record your rating. Repeat these setup statements while tapping on the karate chop point. "Even though I feel apathetic about this, and almost everything, I deeply and completely love and accept all of my feelings, even the ones I'm not yet aware of. Even though I am indifferent to my past, my current situation and my future, I deeply and completely love and accept myself and everything that has led me to this state of apathy. Even though I have somehow managed to suppress all of my emotions, and I can't even get angry or frustrated, I deeply and completely love and accept myself anyway." Repeat a different reminder phrase at each of the eight tapping points.

Eyebrow	I feel apathy
Side of Eye	I even feel apathetic about my apathy
Under the Eye	That's pretty bad, isn't it?
Under the Nose	Even my apathy has apathy
Chin	I don't feel good about that
Collarbone	I don't feel bad about that either

Under the Arm	That is how apathy works
Top of Head	I wonder why I don't feel safe having any feelings?
Eyebrow	Where did I learn that?
Side of Eye	Maybe just one small positive or negative feeling would be okay
Under the Eye	Which feeling feels the safest to me right now?
Under the Nose	What would happen if I dared to feel even one small feeling?
Chin	I acknowledge that my apathy may have helped me feel safe in the past
Collarbone	It used to work well for me
Under the Arm	It may not be working well for me anymore
Top of Head	I am open to receiving messages of clarity about my feelings now

Take a deep breath and let it out. Check the intensity of your original problem statement. "I feel apathetic." Repeat the sequence as needed until the intensity is very low.

People also have different comfort levels with the idea of change. Some people are carefree, and easy spirits that actually are uncomfortable if things remain the same for a very long time. There are other folks that adhere rigidly to schedules and routines and become quite anxious or agitated with even the slightest change. This discomfort around change can persist even if the person is trying to move toward something they really want or need.

Say this problem statement aloud. "I am not comfortable with change." Rate your intensity on the 0-10 point scale. Record your intensity rating. Repeat these setup statements while tapping gently on the karate chop point. "Even though I'm not comfortable with change, and I have never been, I am passionate about wanting things to be different in my life. Change has always felt scary. Even though I don't usually like the result, knowing what to expect, the same old thing, has always felt safer to me than change. In spite of this, I want to love my life. I want to feel excitement and I choose to reclaim my inborn power." Say this reminder phrase at each tapping point.

Eyebrow	I am uncomfortable with change
Side of Eye	I am uncomfortable with change
Under the Eye	I am uncomfortable with change
Under the Nose	I am uncomfortable with change
Chin	I am uncomfortable with change
Collarbone	I am uncomfortable with change
Under the Arm	I am uncomfortable with change
Top of Head	I am uncomfortable with change

Take a deep breath and check the intensity of your original problem statement. "I am not comfortable with change." Record your rating. If your rating is above a 3, continue tapping on the eight points with the reminder phrase until the intensity has decreased. Then, do a round of positive affirmation tapping. Use a different reminder phrase at each of the eight tapping points.

Eyebrow	The past doesn't dictate my future
Side of Eye	Just because change was scary in the past doesn't mean it has to be scary now
Under the Eye	I am passionate about growing and making things better
Under the Nose	Change is a part of that process
Chin	I choose to see change as a powerful ally in my life
Collarbone	My future is mine to create
Under the Arm	Discomfort with change has no place here
Top of Head	I choose to be pleasantly surprised with how I welcome change into my life now

Take a deep breath and let it out. Rate the intensity of your original problem statement. "I am not comfortable with change." Record your rating. Repeat the sequence if you feel continued high intensity.

These examples are not exhaustive but should give you some ideas about how to address the issues that have kept you at the same place in your life, even when you have had the desire to make a change or move forward. If any of the issues have not completely resolved, go back and tap on them again. Feel free to tap without words if the issue is something you can really feel or to change the words to exactly match your situation, thoughts, and feelings.

Psychological Reversal

When I first started learning about meridian tapping, there was a great emphasis placed on psychological reversal. People had lots of different metaphors to explain it. I tend to think of psychological reversal (PR) as a program that causes the opposite reaction from what is expected. Have you ever had the experience of saying that you want to lose weight and then almost immediately you eat a large bowl of ice cream or a candy bar? That is not what you would expect to happen if you say you want to lose weight. It is like there is some internal program running behind the scenes that has control over your behavior and your destiny.

Many people describe this as a spiritual or energetic issue, but no matter how you describe it the result is the same. People that are experincing PR don't have the results they want and often sabotage their own success. Gallo and Vincenzi (2000) describe six different types of self sabotage. These include massive reversal, deep-level reversal, specific reversal, criteria-related reversal, mini-reversal, and recurring reversal. Massive reversals impact most, if not all, of the major areas of life function. Economics, relationships, mood, jobs - they all seem to be chronically going wrong. People experiencing deep-level reversal typically believe that the problem or situation they want to change is bigger or more powerful than they are. Individuals experiencing specific reversal don't have problems in so many different areas of their lives, they have something going on in just one area like a specific phobia.

Criteria-related reversals are another type of reversal in which the problem seems to be specific rather than existing in many life domains. This type commonly involves some sort of thought process or programming that prevents making a change such as shame or guilt. This person often feels unworthy of their desired goal. The fifth type of reversal that Gallo and Vincenzi describe is the mini-reversal. You can think of this as a form of back-sliding. This occurs when you are making progress toward your goal and then stop moving forward or even take a few steps back. Finally, they describe the recurring reversal. Unlike the mini-reversal, this is a return of the problem, going all the way back to the starting line. If you are like me, you have experienced at least two or three of these.

They appear to differ in the ways that they have developed and in the scope of their interference. What these different types have in common is their interference with optimal functioning in your life. Another thing that these different types of PR have in common is that they can be reduced or eliminated using meridian tapping.

The basic tapping procedure that you have already learned usually begins with tapping on the karate chop spot on the side of your hand and saying an admission about the problem and an affirmation about yourself. This is designed to help with PR. You may not have experienced it yet, but people with PR often have a moment of reticence or discomfort when confronted with the statement "I deeply and completely love and accept myself" or any of the other variations of that phrase.

Imagine that you have a deep-level reversal in which you believe that overcoming your food addiction is something that is out of your grasp because it is too big, has too much of a hold on you, and you cannot imagine your life with food being any different than it is now. That's what is going on deep inside, perhaps even at the subconscious level. Then, one day you look in the mirror and say, I'm unhappy with the way I look so I'm going to start my diet tomorrow. Sound familiar? Well, in that moment you really mean it. You just aren't aware that there is a program running in the background called deep-level reversal that is keeping you stuck. Next, a well meaning friend who has heard about this tapping thing suggests you try it. You think - why not? I've tried everything else. Your friend teaches you about the tapping points and you enthusiastically start tapping on your karate chop point, saying "Even though I have this food addiction, I deeply and completely love and accept myself." Those last words are likely to barely come out in a whisper if they come out at all. I have seen people sneeze, choke, cough, or stop dead in their tracks when confronted with saying those words out loud. That is a clue that there is PR at work.

Mini-reversals are also very common when working with food and lifestyle issues. I certainly have experienced many weeks and months of clean, healthy eating only to suddenly find myself standing in the pantry stuffing potato chips in my mouth fast and furiously. When I came to my senses, I was not only mortified to look at how many calories I had just consumed, but also how quickly the reversal came upon me. At first I was completely blindsided and had no idea what the issue was. This change seemed to come out of the blue. After several rounds of tapping I was not only able to identify the issue, but I was able to see solutions as well.

Moving past PR isn't always so easy. Particularly for people with massive reversal, deep-level reversal, and recurring reversal professional help can be useful or even necessary in order to move forward. We don't get this way overnight and we usually have an abundance of help in developing our maladaptive thoughts and behaviors so it makes sense that we might need help to get rid of them as well. Particularly when working with PR, please remember to seek professional assistance if your symptoms seem to be getting worse or if the energy work becomes overwhelming to you.

In addition to tapping on the karate chop point, using setup statements, and using affirmation, there are other ways of addressing PR. There are other tapping points, breathing techniques, and neurolinguistic programming techniques that can be beneficial when working on these issues. Individuals trained in the use of meridian tapping will have lots of ways to help.

A Time for Self-Discovery

What are your main reasons for wanting to change your weight? Your answers will probably be similar to mine and to those of most of your friends. The standard answers include things such as to be healthy, to look good at my next class reunion, so my doctor will get off my back about my weight, and so I can enjoy physical activity more easily. Those are really good answers, but you will have more success if you can be even more specific about your reasons. Look at these examples below.

General Reason	Specific Reason
I want to be healthy	So that my chest doesn't hurt when I climb stairs
To look good at my next class reunion	Because I want to see the look on Joe's face when he realizes what he gave up when he dumped me
So my doctor will get off my back about my weight	To be eager to get on the scales instead of dreading it
So I can enjoy physical activity more easily	So I can fit in the swings when I go to the playground with my children

In your tapping journal or on this page I want you to list your top 10 reasons for wanting to change your weight. Be as specific as you possibly can. Include as much information as it takes for you to get a clear image of what YOU really want. This is not the time to write down things that you think you should want or what other people tell you that they want. This is all about YOU.

1	2
3	4
5	6
7	8
9	10

The next exercise may be a bit more challenging. What is the downside for you in changing your weight? How can there be a downside? I can think of many. Perhaps you are not looking forward to the feelings of deprivation that you are expecting. Maybe you have concerns about the time it might take to prepare healthy meals or to exercise. What about fear of failure? Do you experience panic when considering how you are going to manage your moods if you don't have food to rely upon? It is time to identify at least 10 factors that you would consider the cons or negative side to changing your weight.

1	2
3	4
5	6
7	8
9	10

If someone were to ask you what you get out of being overweight, you might be tempted to punch them. Of course you don't get anything out of being overweight - or do you? Being overweight does have advantages for some people. Our excess weight can serve as a protection from other people or from our own sexuality. Keeping the excess weight also allows us to maintain the status quo rather than risk the possibility of frustration and failure. For some people, being overweight serves as a connection to current family members and to generations that have preceded us. When you hear someone say "All of the women in my family have been heavy" that is a strong statement of identification that could be lost if the individual was to lose weight. These conscious and unconscious benefits of being overweight can have a tremendous impact on your energy system and can be sufficient to stop a weight loss program. Be brutally honest and write down the positive things that are associated with being overweight.

1	2
3	4

5	6
7	8
9	10

Automatic thoughts, often negative, are just that - automatic. They pop into our minds and have a tremendous impact, not only on our current mood but also on our energy system. What thoughts pop into your mind when you hear or think about the words diet, exercise, or weight loss? Write them down in as much detail as you possibly can.

1	2
3	4
5	6
7	8
9	10

What is your emotional or energetic response to the following words, phrases, and statements? Rate each one on the SUDs scale.

I don't deserve to lose weight.	*Rating*	It is not safe for me to lose weight	*Rating*
Deprivation	*Rating*	Failure	*Rating*
I'll just regain the weight	*Rating*	I don't believe I can change	*Rating*
Lonely	*Rating*	Unlovable	*Rating*
Sexy	*Rating*	Security	*Rating*
Expectations	*Rating*	It's too late	*Rating*
I want them to love me for who I am, not what I look like	*Rating*	Sugar Addict	*Rating*
Cravings	*Rating*	Obsessions	*Rating*
Irritable	*Rating*	Anxious	*Rating*
Lazy	*Rating*	Resentment	*Rating*

Each of those words or statements that caused a reaction for you is a potential item that is holding you back from your weight loss success and can be addressed through meridian tapping.

Now you are ready to do some life-changing tapping. When you turn the page you will find a variety of tapping exercises to address cravings, motivation, fears, and random thoughts that I, and many of my clients, have had about food, exercise, and diet. Let's get going.

I have a love-hate relationship with food.

The Setup

Even though I have this love-hate relationship with food, I deeply and completely love and accept myself anyway. Even though I love food, but I hate what it does to my body, I deeply and completely love and accept myself anyway. Even though my relationship with food and with my body is quite problematic for me, I deeply and completely love myself and accept all of these feelings.

The Tapping

Eyebrow	I have a love/hate relationship with food
Side of Eye	This love/hate relationship with food
Under the Eye	I hate what my love of food does to my body
Nose	I love food but I hate my body
Chin	I hate food but I love my body
Collarbone	This love/hate relationship with food
Under the Arm	Even though I have this love/hate relationship with food
Top of Head	I deeply and completely love and accept myself anyway

 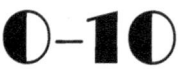 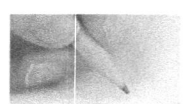

I have trouble thinking about food in a rational way.

The Setup

Even though I have trouble thinking about food in a rational way, I deeply and completely love and accept myself. Even though food is a highly emotional subject for me, I am working toward a different way of relating to food, meals, and eating. Even though I have an emotional reaction to food, I love and accept myself, knowing that I am a work in progress.

The Tapping

Eyebrow	I get irrational about food
Side of Eye	Thinking about food makes me emotional
Under the Eye	Thinking about not having certain foods makes me emotional
Nose	Thinking about limiting certain foods makes me emotional
Chin	Everything about food and eating makes me emotional
Collarbone	And don't say the word diet to me
Under the Arm	I am working on changing these emotional responses
Top of Head	I look forward to seeing food in a new way

   **0-10**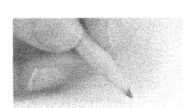

Food is my only friend.

The Setup

Even though it feels sometimes like food is my only friend, I deeply and completely love and accept myself anyway. Even though I eat junk food when I am lonely, and I am afraid of losing my only friend if I stop eating, I choose to find other ways to manage this feeling. Even though it is terrifying to think of changing my relationship with my food/friend, I am open to a new way of being.

The Tapping

Eyebrow	Food is my friend
Side of Eye	How can I give that up?
Under the Eye	Sometimes I think food is my only friend
Nose	I have no idea what I would do instead of eating when I feel lonely
Chin	Even the thought makes me want to eat more
Collarbone	Food feels like my best friend
Under the Arm	Everyone wants a best friend
Top of Head	It's always there when I need it

KEEP GOING TO NEXT PAGE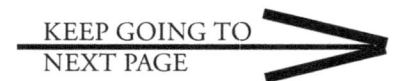

Eyebrow	Food never lets me down
Side of Eye	I always feel better when I eat ice cream or chocolate
Under the Eye	At least for a little while
Nose	Later I feel pretty bad
Chin	I am open to other ways of handling these feelings
Collarbone	Food is just food
Under the Arm	I can learn to handle these feelings in other ways
Top of Head	Feelings are just feelings and I can handle them

 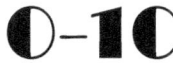 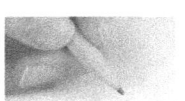

"Treating humans without the concept of energy is treating dead matter!"
- Albert Szent-Gyorgi, M.D., Nobel Prize Laureate

4

I will feel deprived if I cannot eat my favorite foods.

The Setup

Even though I am afraid of how I will feel if I don't eat my favorite foods, I choose to love and accept myself anyway. Even though I am sure I will feel deprived without my favorite foods, I am hopeful that I can find other sources of pleasure in my life. Even though the fear of deprivation is very strong for me, I am beginning to consider small diet changes that will help me to be healthy and happy.

The Tapping

Eyebrow	I feel deprived
Side of Eye	I want to eat my favorite foods
Under the Eye	I don't want to feel deprived
Nose	I need to eat or I will feel deprived
Chin	I will do anything to avoid that feeling
Collarbone	This deprivation
Under the Arm	Fear of deprivation
Top of Head	This strong feeling of deprivation

   **0–10**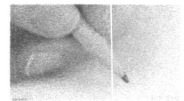

I am afraid I will lose control.

The Setup

Even though I am afraid I will lose control if confronted with any of my favorite foods, I deeply and completely love and accept myself. Even though I am afraid that I will lose control and eat too much or eat foods that are not healthy for me, I choose to focus on loving myself and my healthy body instead. Even though I am afraid that I will lose control and eat like a pig, I choose to feel calm and confident, even when those comfort foods are readily available.

The Tapping

Eyebrow	I am afraid I will lose control
Side of Eye	I am afraid I will eat like a pig
Under the Eye	I am afraid my food plan will go right out the window
Nose	I can't control myself around those foods
Chin	I am afraid I will lose control
Collarbone	I am afraid I will eat too much
Under the Arm	I am afraid I will eat unhealthy foods
Top of Head	I am afraid I will lose control

 **0-10**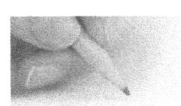

If I exercise now I will be too tired later.

The Setup

Even though I am avoiding exercise right now, I love and accept myself anyway. Even though I am worried that I will be too tired later if I exercise now, I acknowledge that I am a work in progress. Even though I am worried that I will be too tired to do the rest of the things I have planned for my day if I exercise now, I know that I can change this negative way of thinking.

The Tapping

Eyebrow	If I exercise now I will be too tired later
Side of Eye	I am already tired now
Under the Eye	How can I do the things I need to do if I exercise now?
Nose	I know I am just making excuses
Chin	But they have worked for me before
Collarbone	At least they have worked to keep me from exercising
Under the Arm	This excuse hasn't helped me to get any healthier
Top of Head	I know that it isn't even true

KEEP GOING TO NEXT PAGE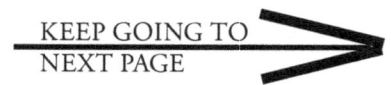

Eyebrow	When I do exercise I am tired for a little while
Side of Eye	And then I have even more energy
Under the Eye	When I exercise regularly
Nose	My energy level stays up
Chin	This is just a negative message my brain has made up
Collarbone	To keep me right where I am
Under the Arm	It isn't a good message
Top of Head	It isn't a true message

 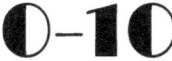 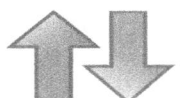

Eyebrow	This is a message I could ignore
Side of Eye	Sometimes my brain tells me things that aren't true
Under the Eye	Things like "I'm hungry" right after I've eaten
Nose	Or things like "If you eat sugar you'll feel better."
Chin	Sometimes these messages are really hard to ignore
Collarbone	I am excited that I can sometimes tell the difference
Under the Arm	I am getting so much better about making decisions based on my goals
Top of Head	I may not be excited about exercising right now, but I don't have to worry about being too tired later

  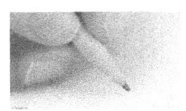

Dieting is just too hard.

The Setup

Even though it feels like dieting is just too hard, I am open to considering baby steps that could make a difference for me. Even though it feels like dieting is just too hard, I choose to remember that I don't have to do it all at once. Even though it feels like dieting is just too hard, I love and accept myself anyway.

The Tapping

Eyebrow	Dieting is just too hard
Side of Eye	I don't want to do anything that is so hard
Under the Eye	It's just too hard
Nose	It seems overwhelming to me
Chin	It's so hard that I don't think I can even face it
Collarbone	Dieting is just too hard
Under the Arm	It's too hard
Top of Head	Dieting is way too hard

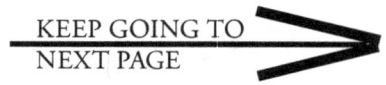

KEEP GOING TO
NEXT PAGE

Eyebrow	Dieting is so very hard
Side of Eye	But I am open to some baby steps toward my goals
Under the Eye	Dieting seems way too hard
Nose	But I don't have to do it all at once
Chin	Dieting is just too hard
Collarbone	I choose to love and accept myself anyway
Under the Arm	I am open to the possibility that it could be easier than I think
Top of Head	I choose to look for the possibility of success

 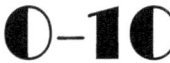 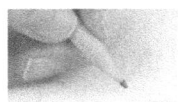

Tapping Exercise:

Think about your first memory involving exercise. How old were you? What did you do? Why? How did it turn out? Were there other people around? What did you see, feel, hear, or taste? Was it a good experience? If not, why? Be as specific as you possibly can. Tap through the usual tapping spots while reflecting on your exercise experience. Write down any thoughts or reactions in response to this exercise in your tapping journal so that you can return to it another time.

8

It is not fair that I have to diet while others eat everything they want.

The Setup

Even though it doesn't feel fair that I have to diet while others eat all of the food they want, I deeply and completely love and accept myself just the way I am. Even though it isn't fair that I have to limit my food in order to get to the weight I desire, I deeply and completely love and accept myself no matter what. Even though other people can eat more than I can and eat different foods than I can, I choose to focus on having the body I really want.

The Tapping

Eyebrow	It's not fair
Side of Eye	It's just not fair
Under the Eye	They can eat anything they want
Nose	I can't
Chin	It's not fair
Collarbone	I want to eat anything I want and still have a great body
Under the Arm	Why them and not me?
Top of Head	It's not fair

   0-10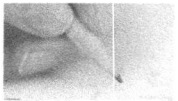

9

Just one bite can't hurt.

The Setup

Just one bite can't hurt me. That's the thought in my head. If I could stop at one bite, it probably would be okay, but I have trouble stopping with just one bite. Even though I am trying to justify eating something that may not be good for me, I deeply and completely love and accept myself anyway. Even though I'm making excuses for eating something that isn't part of my food plan right now, I accept myself, whether I eat that bite or not. I am fighting the impulse to eat, and I am trying to justify my position. I am open to clarity about my feelings, my eating, and this circumstance.

The Tapping

Eyebrow	Just one bite can't hurt me
Side of Eye	One bite won't really matter at all
Under the Eye	I can stop at just one bite
Nose	I can, but I probably won't
Chin	Starting to eat this food may be a bad idea for me right now
Collarbone	I wonder why I want it so badly?
Under the Arm	Do I want the taste of it, or is there something else?
Top of Head	I am open to clarity about these issues

   **0–10**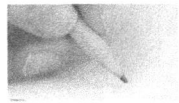

I am afraid to even get started on losing weight.

The Setup

Even though I am afraid to even get started losing weight, I deeply and completely love and accept my feelings and myself. Even though I am afraid to even get started losing weight, I love and accept myself anyway. Even though I am afraid to get started losing weight, I choose to feel calm and confident.

The Tapping

Eyebrow	I am afraid to even get started losing weight
Side of Eye	I am afraid to even get started losing weight
Under the Eye	I am afraid to even get started losing weight
Nose	I am afraid to even get started losing weight
Chin	I am afraid to even get started losing weight
Collarbone	I am afraid to even get started losing weight
Under the Arm	I am afraid to even get started losing weight
Top of Head	I am afraid to even get started losing weight

KEEP GOING TO
NEXT PAGE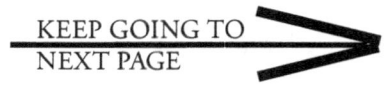

Eyebrow	I have been afraid to even get started losing weight
Side of Eye	It feels good to learn to get over that
Under the Eye	I choose to do what will help me achieve my weight loss goals
Nose	It feels good to actually get started
Chin	I like doing good things for myself
Collarbone	Getting started is behind me now
Under the Arm	I congratulate myself on getting started
Top of Head	I choose to be amazed by how easy it will be now to get to my goal weight

 **0-10**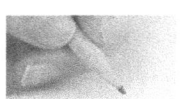

"An early-morning walk is a blessing for the whole day." - Henry David Thoreau

I can't stick to a diet plan, so why start?

The Setup

Even though I can't stick to a diet plan, and I'm not sure it even makes sense to start, I deeply and profoundly love and accept myself and forgive myself for not being able to stick to diet plans in the past. Even though I have difficulty sticking to diets when I start them, and I would rather not start anything than have to live with that failure again, I deeply and profoundly love and accept all of me. Even though sticking to diets has been very difficult for me in the past, and it has been almost impossible, and it has kept me from starting to do anything healthy, I deeply and completely love and accept myself.

The Tapping

Eyebrow	I can't stick to diets
Side of Eye	So why even start?
Under the Eye	It seems ridiculous to even try
Nose	I never stick to it
Chin	I won't stick to it this time either
Collarbone	And you can't make me
Under the Arm	I can't stick to anything
Top of Head	I don't see why I should even start

KEEP GOING TO NEXT PAGE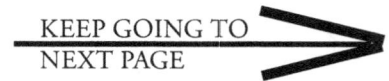

Eyebrow	I determine what I can and cannot do
Side of Eye	I can stick to things when I choose to
Under the Eye	I choose to take positive action in spite of my fear
Nose	This is a new day
Chin	I can start new things
Collarbone	I love myself whether I stick to it or not
Under the Arm	It is my choice
Top of Head	I choose to feel invincible

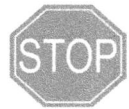 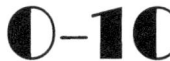 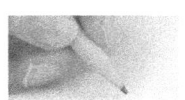

"Get comfortable with being uncomfortable!" - Jillian Michaels

I have strange eating habits.

The Setup

Even though I have strange eating habits, I love and accept myself anyway. Even though I have strange eating habits, I deeply and completely love and accept myself. Even though I have strange eating habits, I love and accept all of me.

The Tapping

Eyebrow	These strange eating habits
Side of Eye	These strange eating habits
Under the Eye	These strange eating habits
Nose	These strange eating habits
Chin	These strange eating habits
Collarbone	These strange eating habits
Under the Arm	These strange eating habits
Top of Head	These strange eating habits

   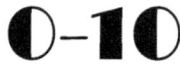   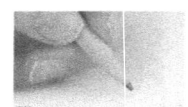

13

I just can't stay fat.

The Setup

I just can't stay fat. The thought of it makes me feel upset. It feels almost like panic. I just can't stay fat. I hate being fat. I don't want to be fat anymore. If I stay fat I won't have any kind of future. I just can't stay fat.

The Tapping

Eyebrow	I can't stay fat
Side of Eye	I can't stay fat
Under the Eye	I can't stay fat
Nose	I can't stay fat
Chin	I can't stay fat
Collarbone	I can't stay fat
Under the Arm	I can't stay fat
Top of Head	I can't stay fat

   **0-10**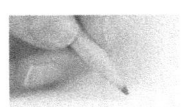

14

I don't know how to stop eating.

The Setup

I don't seem to know how to stop eating. I can have a healthy plan but once I start eating I usually eat too much. I don't understand why I can't just eat a small amount. Leaving food on my plate makes me feel anxious. Leaving food in the saucepan or skillet makes me feel anxious too. I'd like to be able to eat a reasonable portion and then just be done. In spite of all of these frustrations, I choose to love and accept myself anyway.

The Tapping

Eyebrow	I can't stop eating once I start
Side of Eye	I tend to overeat at every meal
Under the Eye	I just can't seem to get enough
Nose	Enough what? I don't know
Chin	I would be lying if I said I was hungry
Collarbone	I rarely eat to stop hunger
Under the Arm	I don't usually get hungry
Top of Head	I eat too much food to really feel hungry

KEEP GOING TO
NEXT PAGE
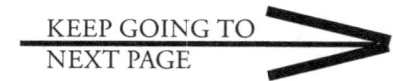

Eyebrow	So why can't I stop eating?
Side of Eye	I plan my meals
Under the Eye	I plan nutritious food
Nose	And then once I start eating I can't seem to stop
Chin	Even though I can't seem to stop eating once I start
Collarbone	I choose to eat according to my plan anyway
Under the Arm	Even though leaving food on my plate makes me feel anxious
Top of Head	I choose to leave food on my plate anyway

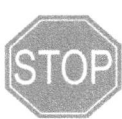 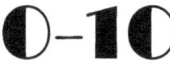 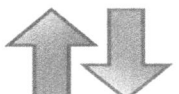

Eyebrow	Even though leaving food in the kitchen makes me feel anxious
Side of Eye	I choose to leave food in the kitchen anyway
Under the Eye	Even though I feel anxious when I don't finish all of the food
Nose	I choose to eat in a healthy way
Chin	All of this food anxiety
Collarbone	I am open to clarity about these confusing feelings
Under The Arm	Food anxiety
Top of Head	I am open to loving myself in spite of all of this confusion

 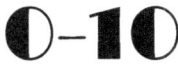 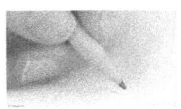

It is bedtime so I need a snack.

The Setup

Even though I feel like I need a snack before bed, I choose to consider the possibility that this is just a habit, not a need. Even though I feel like I need a snack before bed, I choose to address my feelings about bedtime without always turning to food. Even though I feel like I need a snack before bed, I choose to love, honor, and accept myself.

The Tapping

Eyebrow	I always want a bedtime snack
Side of Eye	As soon as I decide it is bedtime
Under the Eye	I automatically start thinking about food
Nose	I've had a bedtime snack
Chin	Since I was a tiny child
Collarbone	It might have made sense for me then
Under the Arm	But I know it doesn't really make sense for me now
Top of Head	Snacks before bed used to make me feel loved and cared for

KEEP GOING TO NEXT PAGE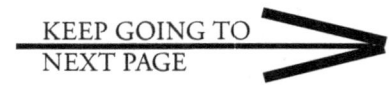

Eyebrow	Now it is just something I do
Side of Eye	My body doesn't need the food so that I can sleep
Under the Eye	In fact, sugary snacks probably interfere with my sleep
Nose	Lets face it
Chin	I love food, and food makes me feel loved
Collarbone	We all want to feel loved
Under the Arm	But I know that food doesn't really do that for me
Top of Head	I am open to more clarity about this issue

 **0-10**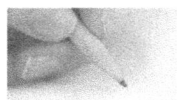

Tapping Exercise:

Stand fully clothed in front of a full length mirror and start tapping. Notice how you look from the front. Turn to your right. What do you see? Turn to your left. What do you see now? Turn your back to the mirror and peek over your shoulder. What did you notice first? Keep tapping and describe your body out loud. Keep looking in the mirror and tapping until you feel comfortable.

16

I am afraid to give up my food pleasure.

The Setup

Even though I am afraid to give up my food pleasure, I deeply and completely love and accept myself. Even though I am afraid to give up my food pleasure, I choose to feed my body with love and logic. Even though I am afraid to give up my food pleasure, I am open to feeling joy and pleasure in other ways.

The Tapping

Eyebrow	I am afraid to give up my food pleasure
Side of Eye	If I give up some of these foods, I may never feel any pleasure ever again
Under the Eye	I have so few pleasures now that I don't want to give any of them up
Nose	What would I ever have to look forward to if I didn't have food?
Chin	I am so afraid to give up my food pleasure
Collarbone	Sometimes it feels like that is all I've got
Under the Arm	I don't think I can give up my food pleasure
Top of Head	Without my food pleasure, there would be no end to my misery

KEEP GOING TO NEXT PAGE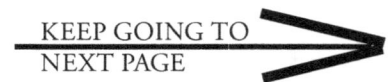

Eyebrow	The pleasure of food keeps the sadness away
Side of Eye	The pleasure of food keeps the boredom away
Under the Eye	The pleasure of food keeps the loneliness away
Nose	I wonder if there is a way to keep some of the pleasure of food
Chin	Without overeating and making myself fat?
Collarbone	That would be a great compromise
Under the Arm	I am open to the small possibility that I don't have to eat so much in order to feel pleasure
Top of Head	I am open to the small possibility that I don't have to eat foods that are bad for my body in order to feel pleasure

 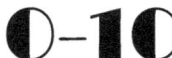 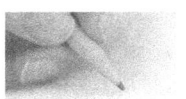

"Energy Medicine is the "Last big frontier
in medicine." - Dr. Mehmet Oz

I can't exercise tonight because I have had a busy day.

The Setup

Even though I don't think I can exercise tonight since I've had such a busy day, I choose to anticipate joy and relief that I am taking good care of my body. Right now I don't think I can exercise because of my busy day, but I reserve the option to re-evaluate in a few minutes when I have taken the time to regroup. Even though I have some excuses about exercising tonight, I choose to consider whether this choice is congruent with my goals or not. I choose to love and accept myself either way.

The Tapping

Eyebrow	I have had a very busy day
Side of Eye	So I don't think I can really exercise tonight
Under the Eye	It would just be too much
Nose	I worked so hard that I deserve to just do nothing for a while
Chin	Just one night off won't really matter
Collarbone	I deserve it
Under the Arm	What am I saying?
Top of Head	Do I deserve to be unhealthy?

KEEP GOING TO
NEXT PAGE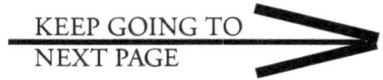

Eyebrow	I love the way I feel after I exercise
Side of Eye	It is true that it doesn't always feel great to get started
Under the Eye	It is true that it sometimes seems pretty hard in the beginning
Nose	I always feel proud of myself when I have the self discipline to exercise
Chin	I could just get started and then quit when my body says it has had enough
Collarbone	If the hectic day means a shorter workout that's okay
Under the Arm	If the hectic day means that a longer workout would be good to help me de-stress, that's okay too
Top of Head	I am open to body guidance about this

   **0-10**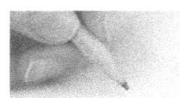

"A bear, however hard he tries, grows tubby without exercise." - A.A. Milne

I feel like giving up.

The Setup

Sometimes I just feel like giving up. Eating right seems too hard. Exercising seems too hard. It all just seems too hard. Even though I feel like giving up, I deeply and completely love and accept myself. Even though I feel like giving up right now, I love and accept myself anyway. Even though I feel like giving up, I choose to demonstrate love and acceptance for myself.

The Tapping

Eyebrow	I feel like giving up
Side of Eye	I feel like giving up
Under the Eye	I feel like giving up
Nose	I feel like giving up
Chin	I feel like giving up
Collarbone	I feel like giving up
Under the Arm	I feel like giving up
Top of Head	I feel like giving up

   **0-10**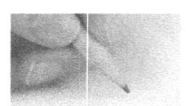

19

I'm not sure I know how to be thin.

The Setup

Being thin has been a goal for so long. I'm not sure how to be a thin person. I know how to lose weight, how to diet, and how to exercise. But then what? I've lived as an obese person for so long that I don't remember what it felt like to be a normal weight. That seems like a lifetime ago. Even though I'm afraid of the unknown associated with being thin, I love and accept my feelings and fears. Even though I am afraid of being thin, I love and accept myself, including my fears. Even though I seem to be afraid, I choose to love and accept myself completely.

The Tapping

Eyebrow	I am afraid of the unknown
Side of Eye	I don't know how to be thin
Under the Eye	I am afraid of the unknown
Nose	I don't like this feeling
Chin	I am afraid of the unknown
Collarbone	And what life would be like as a thin person?
Under the Arm	This seems like a complicated problem for me
Top of Head	And I am open to clarity

 0-10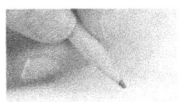

I cannot help it that I am overweight. It is my slow metabolism.

The Setup

Even though I can't help it that I am overweight because I have a slow metabolism, I choose to focus on things I can do to be healthy and active. My metabolism is the problem, not my eating. I can't do anything about that. Can I? I choose to love and accept myself, even my slow metabolism. Even though I can't help it that I am overweight, I choose to love and accept myself just the way I am.

The Tapping

Eyebrow	I can't help it that I am overweight
Side of Eye	Yes, I can
Under the Eye	No, I can't
Nose	I have a slow metabolism
Chin	That makes it hard for me to lose weight
Collarbone	It is very hard
Under the Arm	My metabolism makes it too hard
Top of Head	I can't help it

KEEP GOING TO NEXT PAGE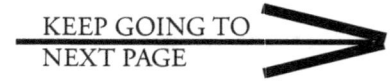

Eyebrow	My metabolism is too slow
Side of Eye	It would be too much work to change that
Under the Eye	I wonder if there are some small things I could do?
Nose	I don't have to do it all today
Chin	I can't help it that I have a slow metabolism
Collarbone	Yes, I can
Under the Arm	I could probably do one or two things differently
Top of Head	I choose to be pleasantly surprised by how easy a few small changes could be

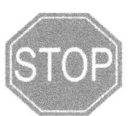 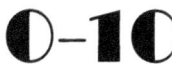 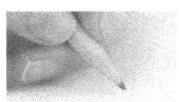

Tapping Exercise:

List 5 food items that evoke strong feelings for you. If you have some of those foods or pictures of those foods, get them out and look at them while you tap. Keep tapping until the feeling is much less intense.

I really want chocolate - NOW!

The Setup

Even though I really want chocolate right now, I deeply and completely love and accept myself anyway. Even though chocolate isn't part of my food plan right now, I acknowledge that I want it anyway. Even though I am craving chocolate right now, I choose to look for other ways to take care of my emotions first. I accept my cravings. I accept my emotions. I am open to clarity.

The Tapping

Eyebrow	I really want chocolate right now
Side of Eye	The craving is very strong
Under the Eye	Chocolate is the only thing that will fix it
Nose	Fix what?
Chin	Chocolate will make me feel better
Collarbone	Chocolate will fix the problem
Under the Arm	I don't even know what the problem is
Top of Head	Then how do I know chocolate is the answer?

KEEP GOING TO
NEXT PAGE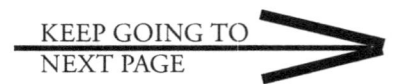

Eyebrow   I am open to clarity about my emotions

Side of Eye   Chocolate won't really fix the problem

Under the Eye   It does taste good

Nose   It is okay to eat chocolate because it tastes good

Chin   I am glad I have tapping to handle these strong cravings

Collarbone   I am in control of my eating

Under the Arm   I can manage my emotions in many ways

Top of Head   I like chocolate but I am learning to love me more

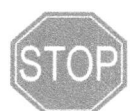   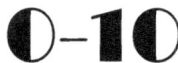   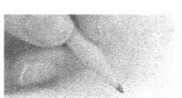

"My grandmother started walking five miles a day when
she was sixty. She's ninety-seven now, and we don't
know where the heck she is." - Ellen DeGeneres

My inner voice says I am not allowed to be thin.

The Setup

Even though my inner voice says I am not allowed to be thin, I deeply and completely love, accept and forgive myself. Even though my inner voice says I am not allowed to be thin, I love and accept myself and all of my feelings. Even though my inner voice says I am not allowed to be thin, I am okay with who I am right now.

The Tapping

Eyebrow	My inner voice says I am not allowed to be thin
Side of Eye	My inner voice says I am not allowed to be thin
Under the Eye	My inner voice says I am not allowed to be thin
Nose	I am not allowed to be thin
Chin	That is what my inner voice keeps saying
Collarbone	My inner voice says I am not allowed to be thin
Under the Arm	I am not allowed to be thin
Top of Head	My inner voice says I am not allowed to be thin

KEEP GOING TO NEXT PAGE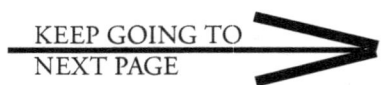

Eyebrow	Wait a minute, I am in charge
Side of Eye	I decide what I can and cannot do
Under the Eye	That wasn't my inner voice talking
Nose	Those were the doubts of everyone else
Chin	Other people's doubts don't make decisions for me
Collarbone	I make decisions for myself
Under the Arm	I am in charge
Top of Head	I am allowed to take care of myself and to be thin

 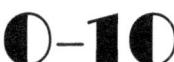 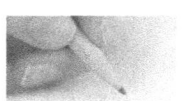

"You only get one body; it is the temple of your soul. Even God is willing to dwell there. If you truly treat your body like a temple, it will serve you well for decades." - Oli Hille

I know I should stop eating so much.

The Setup

I know I should stop eating so much. I don't like how it makes me feel. I don't like how my body looks. It is causing health problems for me. If I am perfrectly honest, I don't want to stop. I can't even say that I want to stop eating without that little voice in my head calling me a liar. I know I don't really mean it. I would like to mean it. So, even though I know I should stop eating so much, and I don't really want to stop, I deeply love, accept, and forgive myself for this internal confusion and choose to feel excited and confident that even this can change for me.

The Tapping

Eyebrow	I know I should stop eating so much
Side of Eye	It's not good for me or my body
Under the Eye	There is a difference between what I know and what I feel
Nose	I am excited to know that even this can change
Chin	I can want to stop eating so much too
Collarbone	I don't need to get hung up on this
Under the Arm	I can tap on this just like I tap on anything else
Top of Head	I can be clear on what it is that I want

0-10

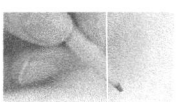

I deserve to have dessert because I have been really good.

The Setup

It makes sense to reward myself with poor health and obesity because I have been good lately. I deeply and completely love and accept myself and that programming. Even though I have bought into that programming in the past and it comes very automatically to me, I am open to new ways of thinking about things. I choose to look for new ways of rewarding myself when dessert isn't the best option. I am open to considering other options when I want an incentive or reward.

The Tapping

Eyebrow	I do deserve to have dessert
Side of Eye	I have been really good
Under the Eye	Dessert can be a fantastic reward for good behavior
Nose	But it isn't the best reward for me right now
Chin	Sometimes dessert is the only reward I can think of
Collarbone	I want to change that
Under the Arm	There are probably other rewards that might feel good.
Top of Head	I am excited to find other ways to honor myself and my body

 **0–10**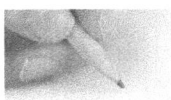

Healthy meals don't stick with me long enough.

The Setup

Healthy meals don't stick with me long enough so I am justified in eating less healthy meals so that I can feel full longer. Even though I have this unhealthy belief, I deeply and completely love and accept myself anyway.

The Tapping

Eyebrow	Healthy meals don't stick with me long enough
Side of Eye	So I have to eat other things to keep me from feeling hungry
Under the Eye	Healthy meals don't stick with me long enough
Nose	So I have to eat other things to keep me from feeling hungry
Chin	Healthy meals don't stick with me long enough
Collarbone	So I have to eat other things to keep me from feeling hungry
Under the Arm	Healthy meals don't stick with me long enough
Top of Head	So I have to eat other things to keep me from feeling hungry

KEEP GOING TO
NEXT PAGE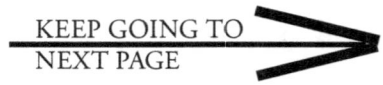

Eyebrow	Healthy meals don't stick with me long enough
Side of Eye	So I have to eat other things to keep me from feeling hungry
Under the Eye	Healthy meals don't stick with me long enough
Nose	So I have to eat other things to keep me from feeling hungry
Chin	Healthy meals don't stick with me long enough
Collarbone	So I have to eat other things to keep me from feeling hungry
Under the Arm	I look forward to replacing this thought with something more reasonable
Top of Head	I choose to change this way of thinking and eating

 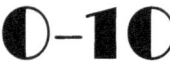 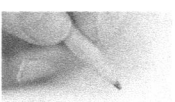

Tapping Exercise:

What was the first negative thing anyone ever said about your body? Start tapping at your eyebrow and continue tapping through the sequence while remembering the event. Imagine that you are viewing the event as a bystander or as if the event were a film clip. Notice every detail. Which parts seem the most important to you? Keep tapping until your distress decreases significantly. Be sure to write down any thoughts or other memories that pop up so that you can tap on them later.

I am so angry about the way my body looks.

The Setup

Even though I feel angry about the way my body looks, I deeply and completely accept myself right now. Even though I feel angry about the way my body looks, I am open to the possibility that I could feel differently about this tomorrow. Even though I feel angry about the way my body looks, I choose to take inspired action.

The Tapping

Eyebrow	I am so angry
Side of Eye	I hate the way my body looks
Under the Eye	And I did this to myself
Nose	I am so angry about the way my body looks
Chin	Doing anything about this feels almost impossible
Collarbone	This anger isn't very healthy for me
Under the Arm	And probably makes it even harder to lose weight
Top of Head	I acknowledge my anger

KEEP GOING TO
NEXT PAGE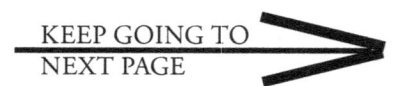

Eyebrow	I acknowledge my challenges
Side of Eye	I accept who I am, even with this less than perfect body
Under the Eye	I have been so angry
Nose	I have been angry about my body's appearance
Chin	And I blame myself for it
Collarbone	That means I've been angry with myself
Under the Arm	I accept where I am right now
Top of Head	And I look forward to a future where I can accept my body too

 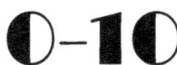 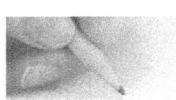

"Thinking about working out burns 0 calories, 0 percentage
of fat and accomplishes 0 goals!" - Gwen Ro

I hate diet shakes and nutrition bars.

The Setup

Even though I hate diet shakes, I choose to love my body. Even though I hate nutrition bars, I choose to focus on my health and well being. Even though I hate diet shakes and nutrition bars, I choose to love and accept myself completely.

The Tapping

Eyebrow	I hate diet shakes
Side of Eye	I hate nutrition bars
Under the Eye	I hate it all
Nose	I want real food
Chin	I don't want diet shakes
Collarbone	I don't want nutrition bars
Under the Arm	Who am I kidding? I don't want real food
Top of Head	I want junk food

KEEP GOING TO NEXT PAGE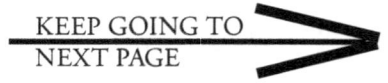

Eyebrow	I don't like the discipline that dieting requires
Side of Eye	Particularly the diet shakes and nutrition bars
Under the Eye	I do have choices
Nose	I don't have to eat anything I don't want to eat
Chin	I could eat real food, healthy food, and reach my goals
Collarbone	Or I can choose the convenience of diet shakes and nutrition bars
Under the Arm	It is really up to me
Top of Head	The choice is up to me

 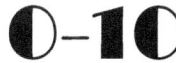 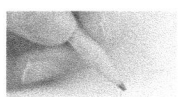

"Typically, people who exercise, start eating better and becoming more productive at work. They smoke less and show more patience with colleagues and family. They use their credit cards less frequently and say they feel less stressed. Exercise is a keystone habit that triggers widespread change." - Charles Duhigg

I'm frustrated.

The Setup

I'm frustrated; not just about one thing, but about many things. I don't like this feeling. I can't seem to fix the things that I'm frustrated about, so I want something sweet and delicious to make me feel better. Even though I am feeling frustrated about all of these things, I choose to manage the real issue, not just cover it up with a sugar high. Even though I am feeling frustrated and just want it to magically go away, I choose to remain open to solutions instead of causing another problem with poor food choices. Even though I really want to eat sweet things right now, I choose to release the frustration instead.

The Tapping

Eyebrow	I'm frustrated
Side of Eye	This frustration
Under the Eye	I'm really feeling frustrated
Nose	I'm frustrated
Chin	This frustration
Collarbone	I want this frustration to just go away
Under the Arm	I'm frustrated
Top of Head	This frustration

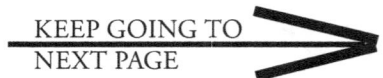

KEEP GOING TO
NEXT PAGE

Eyebrow	I'm so frustrated
Side of Eye	But I am open to seeing options
Under the Eye	I am frustrated
Nose	But I am open to seeking solutions
Chin	I am frustrated
Collarbone	But I choose to allow an easy resolution
Under the Arm	I am frustrated
Top of Head	But I choose to take care of myself without relying on food

 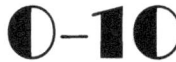 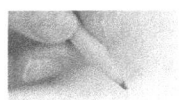

Tapping Exercise:

Start your tapping and remember the first diet you ever started. Be sure to include memories about why you started it, how it went for you, and why you stopped the diet.

29

I want soda.

The Setup

Even though I would really like to drink a soda right now, I love and accept myself. I've decided that soda needs to be a rare treat. I'm struggling with my diet today so it would not be a good day for soda. But I really want it. Why? I suspect that whatever is making me struggle with my diet is also causing me to want the soda. Even though I am craving soda, I am willing to understand this issue more deeply. Even though I am craving soda right now, I acknowledge my feeling as valid, even if I choose not to act on it. Even though I am craving soda right now in response to some feeling I can't even name, I love and accept myself anyway.

The Tapping

Eyebrow	I want a soda
Side of Eye	This soda craving
Under the Eye	I am craving a soda
Nose	I really want a soda
Chin	I'm convinced that it will make me feel better
Collarbone	This soda craving
Under the Arm	My soda craving
Top of Head	I want a soda

KEEP GOING TO NEXT PAGE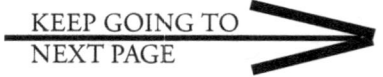

Eyebrow	I really want a soda
Side of Eye	I have a powerful soda craving
Under the Eye	I'd like to drink a soda
Nose	I really want a soda
Chin	My soda craving
Collarbone	I want a soda to make me feel better
Under the Arm	Soda craving
Top of Head	This soda craving

   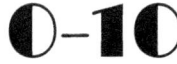   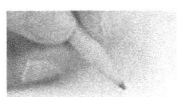

"To resist the frigidity of old age, one must combine the body, the mind, and the heart. And to keep these in parallel vigor one must exercise, study, and love." - Charles-Victor De Bonstettin

Food is my only pleasure.

The Setup

Even though it feels like food is my only pleasure, I love and accept myself anyway. Even though it feels like food is my only pleasure right now, I deeply and completely love and accept myself anyway. Even though it sometimes feels like food is my only pleasure, I love and accept myself and all of my thoughts, feelings, and behaviors related to this issue.

The Tapping

Eyebrow	Food is my only pleasure
Side of Eye	And I don't want to give it up
Under the Eye	Food is my only pleasure
Nose	And I don't want to give it up
Chin	Food is my only pleasure
Collarbone	And I don't want to give it up
Under the Arm	Food is my only pleasure
Top of Head	And I don't want to give it up

   **0-10**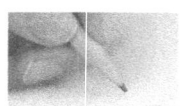

I feel shame about my eating.

The Setup

Even though I feel ashamed about my eating, I choose to love and accept myself anyway. Even though I feel ashamed about my eating, I choose to love and accept myself unconditionally. Even though I feel ashamed about my eating, I deeply and completely love and accept myself.

The Tapping

Eyebrow	This eating shame
Side of Eye	This eating shame
Under the Eye	This eating shame
Nose	This eating shame
Chin	This eating shame
Collarbone	This eating shame
Under the Arm	This eating shame
Top of Head	This eating shame

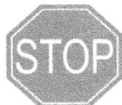 0–10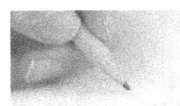

I have a big appetite.

The Setup

Even though I have a big appetite, I love and accept myself. Even though I have a big appetite, I deeply and completely love and accept myself. Even though I have a big appetite, and that is why I eat so much, I love and accept myself anyway.

The Tapping

Eyebrow	I have a big appetite
Side of Eye	That's why I eat so much
Under the Eye	It's not my fault
Nose	If you have a big appetite
Chin	You have to eat lots of food
Collarbone	What does it mean to have a big appetite?
Under the Arm	It's probably just another way to say that I eat too much
Top of Head	It sounds like an excuse

KEEP GOING TO
NEXT PAGE
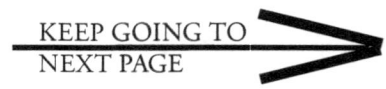

Eyebrow	I choose to be done with excuses
Side of Eye	I do have a big appetite right now
Under the Eye	But I am open to having a smaller one in the future
Nose	I have had a big appetite in the past
Chin	And look where that has led me
Collarbone	I choose to exercise control over my eating
Under the Arm	Whether I have a big appetite or not
Top of Head	I choose to remain in control of my appetite and my food choices

 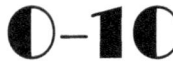 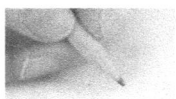

Tapping Exercise:

Spend some time reflecting on meals that occurred during your childhood. Were these generally happy times, stressful times, or really awful times? Were there meals that stand out for you? Tap about the events that were traumatic for you.

I feel lonely. Bring on the food.

The Setup

I feel like eating and that doesn't make a lot of sense. I just finished supper. This strong desire for food has to be about something other than hunger. I think what it is really about is loneliness. I'm not feeling very close to people right now. Food doesn't disappoint me the way people can. Food doesn't leave me alone like people sometimes have. Food is always there for me, so I turn to food when I am lonely. Even though I am using food to soothe my loneliness, I love and accept myself and my feelings. Even though I am feeling lonely right now, I choose to seek real solutions rather than turn to food. Even though I am feeling lonely right now, I choose to release the anger, resentment, and frustration that I am holding inside me.

The Tapping

Eyebrow	I feel lonely
Side of Eye	So bring on the food
Under the Eye	I don't like feeling lonely
Nose	And I want the feeling to go away
Chin	Right now!
Collarbone	This loneliness
Under the Arm	This deep loneliness that fills me up
Top of Head	I feel lonely

KEEP GOING TO NEXT PAGE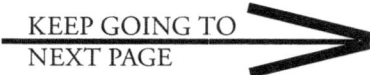

Eyebrow	Feeling lonely seems unacceptable to me
Side of Eye	I could choose to just feel it and let it pass
Under the Eye	But instead, I want to eat
Nose	I'm not talking about celery either
Chin	I'm more interested in calling all of my food friends to be with me
Collarbone	Like chocolate, cookies, cakes, and anything sugary
Under the Arm	Those friends never let me down
Top of Head	At least that is the way I am feeling right now

 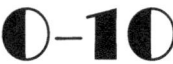 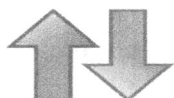

Eyebrow	Even though I am feeling lonely right now
Side of Eye	I choose to look for options
Under the Eye	I am open to clarity
Nose	I feel lonely right now
Chin	But food can't really change my people relationships
Collarbone	It just changes my level of awareness
Under the Arm	Turning to food to ease my loneliness
Top of Head	Will only make me feel worse in the long run

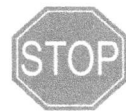 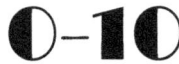 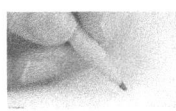

Exercise feels like work.

The Setup

Exercise feels like work and I already work too much. It is hard to even think about working more. I just want to relax and have fun. I know my body needs more exercise. I've been feeling very resistant. Even though I've been resisting exercise because it feels too much like work, I love and accept myself anyway. Even though I am rejecting exercise because it feels too much like work, I love and accept myself anyway. Even though exercise seems like a lot of work, and I'm already overwhelmed, I choose to love myself enough to do what is good for me.

The Tapping

Eyebrow	Exercise feels like work to me
Side of Eye	At least that is my current excuse
Under the Eye	In reality, I'm just upset about how hard I seem to be working
Nose	And I sound just a little resentful about that
Chin	It doesn't make sense to reject exercise because of resentment
Collarbone	Avoiding exercise isn't going to make my work go away
Under the Arm	In reality, exercise is going to make the rest of my work go better
Top of Head	The problem isn't the exercise

KEEP GOING TO
NEXT PAGE
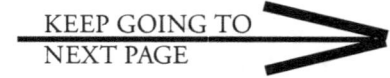

Eyebrow	It is the way I've been thinking about it
Side of Eye	I am open to learning better ways to handle all of the work I am doing
Under the Eye	So that it will be easier to find time to exercise
Nose	I am open to clarity about my resentment
Chin	So that I can learn to enjoy exercise more fully
Collarbone	I choose to address the real life issues
Under the Arm	Instead of making excuses not to exercise
Top of Head	I look forward to a time when exercise is something I want to do instead of something I avoid

 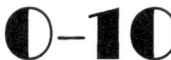 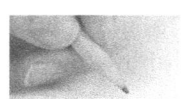

"I am a better person when I have less on my plate." - Elizabeth Gilbert

I don't overeat because of emotions. I overeat because I love food.

The Setup

I don't think that emotional eating is my problem. I eat because I love food and there is so much delicious food out there. I enjoy thinking about food, preparing food, and eating food. I don't see how that can be bad, until I look in the mirror. I would like to learn how to eat the food I love without overeating. Even though I overeat when I get the chance to eat good food, I choose to love and accept myself. Even though I overeat, I would like to love and accept myself anyway. Even though I overeat when I get the chance to eat good food, I am open to seeing this in a new way.

The Tapping

Eyebrow	I overeat
Side of Eye	I don't believe it is because of emotions
Under the Eye	I think I overeat because I love food
Nose	Either way, I still overeat
Chin	And that is not good for me
Collarbone	I would like to learn to eat just what my body needs
Under the Arm	I still want to enjoy good food
Top of Head	I am open to seeing this in a new way

KEEP GOING TO NEXT PAGE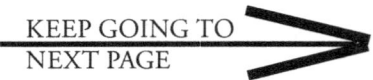

Eyebrow	Eating good food does make me feel good
Side of Eye	And feeling good is an emotion
Under the Eye	I could acknowledge that I want to feel good
Nose	And food is one way to do that
Chin	I am glad that I enjoy good food
Collarbone	I am thrilled that there is so much good food available
Under the Arm	Food can be fun
Top of Head	I choose to enjoy food, but in moderation

   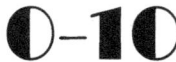   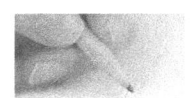

"Your body has the ability to heal itself." - Andrew Weil, M.D.

Losing the same 5 pounds over and over again is really depressing.

The Setup

Even though I've lost this same 5 pounds before, I choose to be amazed at how easy it will be to keep it off this time. Even though I've lost this same 5 pounds before, I respect my choice to lose it again. Even though I've lost this same 5 pounds before, I love and accept myself anyway.

The Tapping

Eyebrow	I am so depressed
Side of Eye	Because I've lost the same 5 pounds before
Under the Eye	Not just once
Nose	But over and over again
Chin	That feels like failure to me
Collarbone	I know it doesn't have to keep happening that way
Under the Arm	But it feels like this cycle will never stop
Top of Head	I acknowledge my frustration

KEEP GOING TO
NEXT PAGE
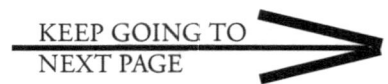

Eyebrow	I acknowledge that I am feeling bad about this
Side of Eye	I don't want to continue the struggle
Under the Eye	I would like to find a way to make this easier
Nose	Stressing out over it won't help me reach my goal
Chin	I am proud of myself for not giving up
Collarbone	I'd like to keep it off this time
Under the Arm	And I am open to having it be much easier
Top of Head	I love and accept myself, with or without this struggle

 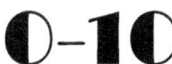 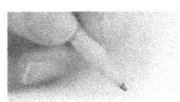

Tapping Exercise:

Look at your stomach. Take a really good look at it from the front, from the side, clothed, and naked. What are the first words or thoughts that pop into your mind? Tap about those.

I can't be happy if I don't lose weight.

The Setup

I just can't be happy if I don't lose weight. I blame my weight for all of the unhappiness in my life and I need it to all go away. I accept all of my feelings about this. I accept all of my thoughts about this. I am open to learning to love and accept myself more.

The Tapping

Eyebrow	I can't be happy if I don't lose weight
Side of Eye	I can't love myself like I am now
Under the Eye	I am so ashamed of my fat
Nose	I cannot accept myself because of how I look
Chin	I worry about what other people think of me too
Collarbone	How can I be happy if I don't lose weight?
Under the Arm	I can't be happy if I don't lose weight
Top of Head	I just can't be happy if I don't lose the weight

   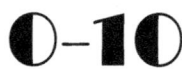   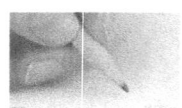

I just want something sweet.

The Setup

Even though I really want something sweet to eat right now, I love and accept myself completely. That includes my sweet tooth. Even though I really want something sweet to eat, I'm still an okay person. Even though I really want something sweet right now, I choose to remain calm and rational.

The Tapping

Eyebrow	I want something sweet right now
Side of Eye	I'm not really hungry
Under the Eye	I just want something sweet
Nose	I have always had a sweet tooth
Chin	A meal doesn't feel complete without something sweet
Collarbone	Unfortunately, fruit doesn't usually make this feeling go away
Under the Arm	At least it hasn't in the past
Top of Head	I want something sweet right now

0–10

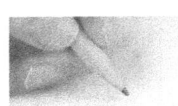

There's nothing to eat.

The Setup

Even though it seems like there is nothing to eat in my kitchen right now, I choose to remain open to the possibilities. Even though it seems like there is nothing to eat in my pantry right now, I accept my thoughts and feelings about this. Even though it seems like there is nothing to eat in my house right now so I'm sure I should go out to eat, I love and accept myself anyway.

The Tapping

Eyebrow	There's nothing to eat
Side of Eye	I am hungry and there is nothing to eat
Under the Eye	I am tired and there is nothing to eat
Nose	I am frustrated and there is nothing to eat
Chin	I know I am being irrational because I see lots of cans, bottles, and jars in my pantry
Collarbone	I know I am being irrational because I see food in my refrigerator
Under the Arm	But I still feel like there is nothing to eat
Top of Head	I could be more accurate and say that I don't see anything that I feel like cooking right now

KEEP GOING TO NEXT PAGE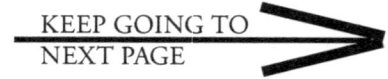

Eyebrow	I could say that I am frustrated because I didn't plan ahead
Side of Eye	I could say that I am struggling to come up with a dinner plan right now
Under the Eye	Those statements would be more accurate and maybe would lead to a solution
Nose	I choose to be more accurate with my thoughts and self statements about food
Chin	Saying that there is nothing to eat would only increase my anxiety
Collarbone	I don't need more anxiety in my life
Under the Arm	Particularly when it isn't even true
Top of Head	I choose to relax and think about this more calmly

 **0–10**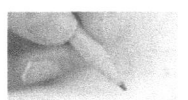

"Energy psychology is entering the mainstream not only
due to its efficiency, but also due to the great need
that exists throughout society." - Fred P. Gallo

That chocolate chip cookie smells so good.

The Setup

Even though that chocolate chip cookie smells so good, I love and accept myself anyway. Even though that warm chocolate chip cookie smells so good, and it is making my mouth water, I love and accept myself anyway. Even though that warm gooey chocolate chip cookie smells so wonderful, I love and accept myself completely.

The Tapping

Eyebrow	That chocolate chip cookie smells so good
Side of Eye	It is making my mouth water
Under the Eye	I can't believe he is eating that right next to me
Nose	The smell is making me feel crazy and out of control
Chin	I really wish everyone would stop eating yummy things
Collarbone	That would make my life so much easier
Under the Arm	I know I won't eat that cookie because of my allergies
Top of Head	But I could go eat something else that might be yummy

KEEP GOING TO NEXT PAGE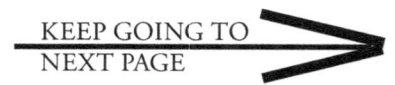

Eyebrow	I want to find something that could make me feel as good as I think that yummy cookie could
Side of Eye	I am really afraid that I am going to give in to this craving
Under the Eye	Smell is a really powerful trigger for me
Nose	In spite of this, I choose to remain calm and confident
Chin	That cookie smells so very, very good
Collarbone	That does not mean that I have to eat it
Under the Arm	I could just enjoy the smell
Top of Head	Now that is a new thought - and I love it!

 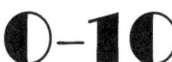 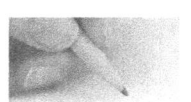

"No one wakes up in the morning and says, I want to gain 150 pounds and I will start right now- Tricia Cunningham

I deserve to eat on my birthday.

The Setup

Even though I feel entitled to overeat on my birthday, I choose to keep my goals in mind. Even though I feel that I really deserve to blow my diet since it is a special occasion, I choose to find ways to celebrate without hurting my health. Even though there is a possibility that I will "blow it," I deeply and completely accept myself, including the parts of me that want indulgence.

The Tapping

Eyebrow	It's my birthday
Side of Eye	I deserve to eat whatever I want
Under the Eye	It doesn't seem fair to have to say no to food on my birthday
Nose	I want steak or lobster
Chin	I want cake and ice cream
Collarbone	I want pancakes and bacon for breakfast
Under the Arm	How can my day be special without those things?
Top of Head	Of course I could eat all of that but just eat smaller portions

KEEP GOING TO NEXT PAGE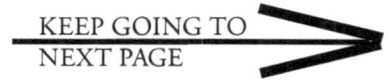

Eyebrow	But I'm not sure that would satisfy me either
Side of Eye	Shouldn't I be able to have whatever I want on my birthday?
Under the Eye	The answer is yes. But, maybe I should look closer at what I really want
Nose	Will those foods make me feel good about myself?
Chin	No they won't
Collarbone	Will overeating make me feel loved?
Under the Arm	No it won't
Top of Head	I choose to find ways to love myself on my birthday without hurting my health

 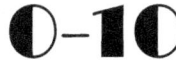 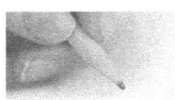

Tapping Exercise:

Name 3 comfort foods. While tapping through the points, describe them in as much detail as you possibly can. Continue tapping while you describe your first memory of these foods. Spend some time thinking about what these foods mean to you, when you crave them the most, and how you feel when you eat them.

I hate situps.

The Setup

I really hate situps. They say that working on our core is crucial to having good health. I just can't seem to make myself do them. Even though I really hate situps and I rarely do any core strengthening exercises, I choose to love and accept myself anyway. Even though I have definitely neglected my core I deeply and completely love and accept that part of myself that is at least trying to do what my body needs. Even though I really hate situps, I choose to be amazed by how easy they could seem in the future.

The Tapping

Eyebrow	I hate situps
Side of Eye	I really hate situps
Under the Eye	They are so hard for me
Nose	I know that strengthening my core muscles would be a good thing
Chin	I know that doing situps and other exercises would help me lose even more weight
Collarbone	But I have been unable to make myself do them in the past
Under the Arm	What if there is a way to actually feel good about doing them?
Top of Head	What if they don't have to be awful?

KEEP GOING TO NEXT PAGE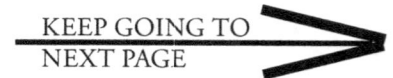

Eyebrow	I could focus on how good those muscles feel to actually receive some attention
Side of Eye	I could focus on how my waist measurement is changing as I am faithful with my workouts
Under the Eye	I could use my situp time to acknowledge everything that I have to be grateful for
Nose	I could use my situp time to send positive energy to situations and people that are important to me
Chin	I am starting to feel a little bit more positive about working on my core muscles
Collarbone	I am starting to feel a little bit more confident in my ability to do situps
Under the Arm	It really wouldn't add that much more time to my workout
Top of Head	And I am excited to think that this workout will make me look even better

 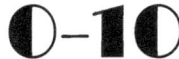 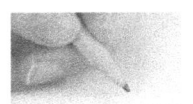

"True discipline is really just self-remembering; no forcing or fighting is necessary." - Charles Eisenstein

I might as well eat whatever I want because I already blew it.

The Setup

I already blew my diet so I might as well eat whatever I want. There's no point in controlling my food now. I've already pointed the guilt finger at myself. I'm already wallowing in blame. So I might as well eat. Even though all of these things are true, I want to love and accept myself anyway. It's pretty hard to love and accept myself with all of this guilt and shame, but I am open to the possibility that I could learn to do it. Even though I am a quitter and planning to give up immediately just because I slipped off of my food plan, I want to choose to start again right now.

The Tapping

Eyebrow	I already blew it
Side of Eye	I already ate something that is on my forbidden list
Under the Eye	I ate way too much of it too
Nose	I feel the guilt and shame
Chin	I might as well go ahead and eat whatever I want
Collarbone	That is what quitters do
Under the Arm	I am a guilty and shameful quitter
Top of Head	Ouch. That smarts.

KEEP GOING TO NEXT PAGE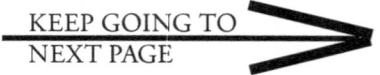

Eyebrow	Sometimes I give up
Side of Eye	Sometimes I don't
Under the Eye	I don't have to give up just because I made a mistake
Nose	I have options
Chin	I have choices
Collarbone	I already blew it might not be totally accurate
Under the Arm	I wouldn't tell anyone else to give up just because of a simple error
Top of Head	I am not going to tell myself that right now either. I can start back on my food plan whenever I choose, including now

   **0-10**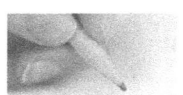

"It is easier to change a man's religion than to change his diet." - Margaret Mead

I look terrible.

The Setup

Even though I look terrible with all of the extra weight, I am trying to keep a positive outlook. Even though I feel hopeless about ever looking any better, what have I really got to lose? Even though I think I look fat and ugly at this point in my life, it hasn't always been this way and it doesn't have to be this way in the future.

The Tapping

Eyebrow	Being overweight and losing weight makes me look terrible
Side of Eye	I will never be able to lose all of this weight
Under the Eye	I have got to begin somewhere
Nose	It won't hurt to try
Chin	I can never lose enough weight to look decent
Collarbone	I know other people have been successful in losing weight, so why can't I?
Under the Arm	I am losing weight slowly and steadily
Top of Head	Certainly if I keep this up, over the next 6 months, I will lose at least 25 pounds or more

   **0-10**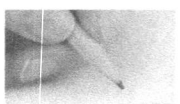

I'm so frustrated that I let myself gain weight again.

The Setup

My weight is back up and that is really frustrating. You would think that I would have gotten control of this by now. I've done this so many times. Even though I'm very frustrated with myself right now, I am learning to love and accept myself anyway. Even though my weight is up, I choose to remember that I've lost weight successfully before. Even though I'm frustrated with my up again, down again weight roller coaster, I choose to keep working toward my health and fitness goals.

The Tapping

Eyebrow	I am frustrated with my weight gain
Side of Eye	I am frustrated with my weight gain
Under the Eye	I am frustrated with my weight gain
Nose	I am frustrated with my weight gain
Chin	I am frustrated with my weight gain
Collarbone	I am frustrated with my weight gain
Under the Arm	I am frustrated with my weight gain
Top of Head	I am frustrated with my weight gain

 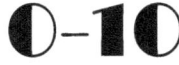 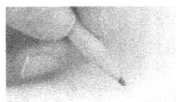

Holidays are all about the food.

The Setup

Every time I think about the holidays I get images of food. I wish I didn't. I would much prefer to associate holidays with something other than food. Even though I have this unwanted association between holidays and food, I choose to love myself anyway. Even though I have this unwanted association between holidays and food, I choose to accept my feelings anyway. Even though I have these unwanted associations between the holidays and food, I choose to accept myself anyway and to remember that I am a work in progress.

The Tapping

Eyebrow	Food and holiday celebrations go together
Side of Eye	If you took the food away I don't know what would be left
Under the Eye	Unfortunately, most holiday foods aren't very good for me
Nose	And overeating seems to be the norm
Chin	It doesn't feel like the holiday without cheesy goodness
Collarbone	It is not a real holiday without cookies and candies
Under the Arm	It doesn't feel like the holiday without appetizers and snacks
Top of Head	There has been so much focus on the food that I don't know what else to do

KEEP GOING TO NEXT PAGE
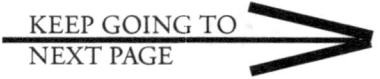

Eyebrow	Even though food equals holiday for me
Side of Eye	I choose to look for new symbols to make myself feel good
Under the Eye	Even though I seem to have always focused on the food
Nose	I choose to focus more on the people and relationships
Chin	Even though food has always been a huge part of the holiday for me
Collarbone	I choose to find other ways to have fun
Under the Arm	I am afraid that without the food it just won't seem right
Top of Head	But I choose to find other ways to celebrate

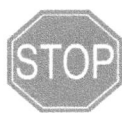 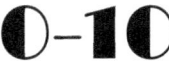 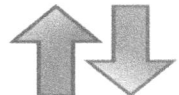

Eyebrow	I love and accept my thoughts about this
Side of Eye	I love and accept my feelings about this
Under the Eye	I love and accept my willingness to learn new ways of celebrating
Nose	I am open to clarity about my relationship with food
Chin	I am open to clarity about my relationship with the holidays
Collarbone	I choose to enjoy food
Under the Arm	Without making it the most important part of the holiday
Top of Head	I am excited about improving my holiday celebrations

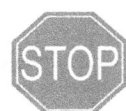 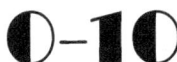 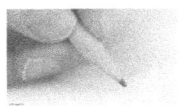

I have a headache. I must need to eat.

The Setup

Even though I have this headache, I deeply and completely love and accept myself. My first thought when I have a headache is that I need to eat. Even though this is my thought, I love and accept myself anyway. Even though I have this headache, I am open to the possibility that something other than food may be the answer.

The Tapping

Eyebrow	I have a headache
Side of Eye	I don't like headaches
Under the Eye	When I have a headache I turn to food
Nose	When I have a headache I want comfort
Chin	I seem to have food and comfort confused
Collarbone	I want my headache to go away
Under the Arm	I haven't even tried anything else
Top of Head	I haven't even looked for reasons that I have a headache

KEEP GOING TO NEXT PAGE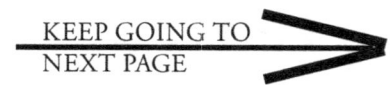

Eyebrow	I am reacting rather than solving my problem
Side of Eye	It is true that sometimes food does work
Under the Eye	But the truth is that it sometimes makes it worse
Nose	I choose to solve my problem rather than eating
Chin	I will feel so much worse about myself if I eat too much
Collarbone	I have a headache
Under the Arm	I have many options for dealing with it
Top of Head	I choose to remain faithful to my food plan

 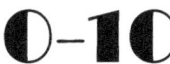 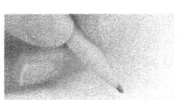

"It is valuable for one to periodically check his/her mindset or system of beliefs to see if it is still operationally valid." - William Tiller, Ph.D.

No matter how hard I work, nothing changes.

The Setup

No matter how hard I work, nothing seems to change. I am frustrated by how little success I have had, no matter how hard I work at it. I accept this frustration as a natural consequence of life. Even though it seems that my hard work doesn't really pay off, I choose to love and accept myself anyway. Even though nothing seems to change, I choose to remember that I have options.

The Tapping

Eyebrow	I work really hard
Side of Eye	But nothing seems to change
Under the Eye	I have always worked very hard
Nose	But where are the results to show for it?
Chin	I diet
Collarbone	But I am still fat
Under the Arm	I exercise
Top of Head	But I am still fat

KEEP GOING TO
NEXT PAGE
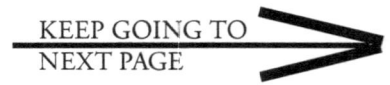

Eyebrow	No matter how hard I try
Side of Eye	Nothing seems to really change
Under the Eye	That goes against my view of how things are supposed to be
Nose	Work hard - get great results
Chin	That's the way things are supposed to be
Collarbone	I acknowledge my frustration
Under the Arm	I acknowledge my disappointment
Top of Head	I am tired of feeling this way

   **0-10**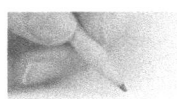

Tapping Exercise:

Look at your thighs. Take a really good look at them from the front, from the side, clothed, and naked. What are the first words or thoughts that pop into your mind? Tap about those.

49

I feel too overwhelmed to get healthy right now.

The Setup

Even though I feel too overwhelmed right now to get healthy, and that is my excuse for not tapping, I deeply and completely love and accept myself and all of my feelings - even my excuses. Even though I feel too overwhelmed right now to get healthy, I deeply and completely love and accept all of me anyway. Even though I have been too overwhelmed in the past to get healthy, I am open to seeing things change for me very soon.

The Tapping

Eyebrow	I feel overwhelmed
Side of Eye	So I can't tap
Under the Eye	I feel overwhelmed
Nose	So overwhelmed that I can't even do anything; certainly not healthy things
Chin	I can't even tap because I'm so overwhelmed
Collarbone	I feel overwhelmed
Under the Arm	I AM overwhelmed
Top of Head	You would be too if you were me

KEEP GOING TO NEXT PAGE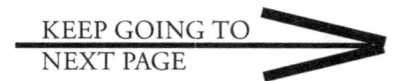

Eyebrow	I have good reasons to feel overwhelmed
Side of Eye	I am overwhelmed and I can't get healthy right now
Under the Eye	It's okay if I'm stuck
Nose	Well, maybe its not okay with me
Chin	I could probably tap
Collarbone	Even though I am so overwhelmed
Under the Arm	And I feel pretty good after I tap
Top of Head	It just might work

 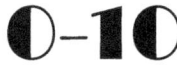 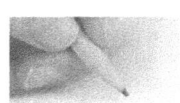

"No disease that can be treated by diet should be treated with any other means." - Maimonides

I do not think I have the willpower for dieting.

The Setup

Even though I don't think I have the willpower for dieting, I deeply and completely love and accept myself anyway. Even though I don't think I have the willpower for dieting, I deeply and completely love and accept myself. I love and accept myself, even though I don't have any willpower.

The Tapping

Eyebrow	I don't think I have the willpower
Side of Eye	I don't think I have what it takes
Under the Eye	Whatever that is
Nose	I don't think I have the willpower for dieting
Chin	What is the point in doing this if I don't have the willpower?
Collarbone	We're jumping way ahead here if I don't even have that
Under the Arm	I don't have any willpower
Top of Head	I know I don't have the willpower to do this

KEEP GOING TO NEXT PAGE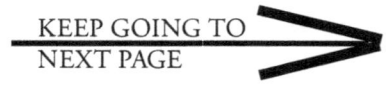

Eyebrow	I have lots of skills and sometimes I have willpower
Side of Eye	I have accomplished many things
Under the Eye	I could probably do this, even without willpower
Nose	I can use all of my skills and learn some new ones too
Chin	There are always people who can teach me things
Collarbone	I can rely on others if my willpower fails me
Under the Arm	I can improve my willpower if I need to because it is just a skill
Top of Head	I have everything I really need

   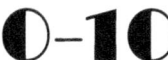   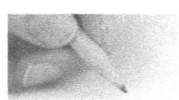

Tapping Exercise:

What do you believe would be your perfect weight? While you are tapping through the points, think about your ideal weight. When was the last time you were at that weight? What was going on in your life? How did you feel? What do you believe is preventing you from weighing that now?

51

I cannot see myself being any different.

The Setup

Even though I can't see myself being any different, I choose to remain open to new possibilities, even weight loss. Even though I can't see myself being any different, I choose to trust that there are good things in my future. Even though I can't see myself being any different, I choose to borrow confidence from other people so that I can anticipate the success of reaching my goal weight.

The Tapping

Eyebrow	I can't see my body being any different
Side of Eye	I have to see it to believe it
Under the Eye	That is just the kind of person I am
Nose	Seeing is believing
Chin	But I just can't see it
Collarbone	I never do anything if I can't see it first
Under the Arm	I can see the grocery store when I leave my house to go to it
Top of Head	I can see the beach before I leave on vacation

KEEP GOING TO
NEXT PAGE

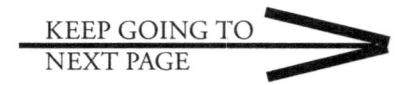

Eyebrow	No I can't
Side of Eye	That is silly
Under the Eye	But this is different
Nose	Why is it different?
Chin	It just feels different
Collarbone	I'm being stubborn
Under the Arm	I prefer to see things before I do them
Top of Head	When I believe the destination exists I can move forward more easily

 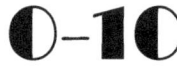 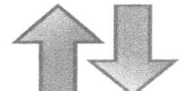

Eyebrow	That seems normal to me
Side of Eye	Seeing is believing
Under the Eye	And believing can be seeing
Nose	I choose to see myself being different
Chin	I believe my body can be different
Collarbone	I know it can be different
Under the Arm	I don't have to see it first
Top of Head	I already know it is there

 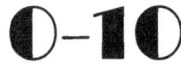 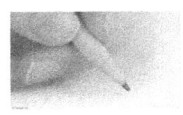

I am PMSing so I have to eat.

The Setup

I have PMS and that usually means I feel ravenous. The only thing that works for my PMS is to eat. If I don't, you don't want to know what I might do. Food usually keeps me calm when I have PMS and I don't know what would do if I didn't gorge myself right now. That is somewhat scary. I deeply love and accept myself even though I feel so out of control right now. Even though I am out of control with PMS, I choose to remember that this is only temporary and I will get through it somehow. Even though this PMS thing is very strong for me, I can choose to deal with it in other ways.

The Tapping

Eyebrow	I have PMS
Side of Eye	I have PMS
Under the Eye	I have PMS
Nose	That means I need to eat
Chin	That means I need to eat whatever I want
Collarbone	I need to eat how much I want of whatever I want right now
Under the Arm	Don't be silly. No it doesn't. I still have choices
Top of Head	I choose to eat sensibly, even though I have PMS

   **0-10**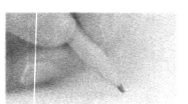

The last five pounds are always impossible.

The Setup

No one ever loses those last few pounds. It doesn't really matter what you do, they just don't seem to go away. You can ask anyone. The first pounds come off easy, but the last few pounds just stick around forever. I might as well give up. Even though I'm considering giving up on the last five pounds since they are always impossible, I am trying to hold onto just a little bit of hope. Even though these last five pounds don't seem like they will ever come off, I choose to love and accept myself anyway.

The Tapping

Eyebrow	I can't ever seem to lose the last five pounds
Side of Eye	Why even try?
Under the Eye	In fact, I might as well give in and eat what I want
Nose	I'm just not meant to get to my goal
Chin	Those last few pounds will stick around forever
Collarbone	Those last five pounds don't seem like they will ever come off
Under the Arm	I can't lose the last five pounds
Top of Head	I won't ever be able to reach my goal

 **0-10**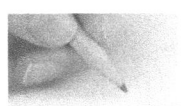

I have a sluggish metabolism.

The Setup

Even though I have a sluggish metabolism, and I don't believe that there is anything I can do about that, I deeply and completely love and accept myself, sluggish metabolism and all. Even though I have a sluggish metabolism that makes it almost impossible for me to reach my goals, I deeply and completely love and accept all of me. Even though I have a sluggish metabolism that causes me to pack on fat quickly, I deeply and completely love and accept myself, just as I am right now.

The Tapping

Eyebrow	I have a sluggish metabolism
Side of Eye	I am carb sensitive
Under the Eye	And I pack on fat quickly
Nose	That means I can never make a mistake
Chin	I have to be extra perfect
Collarbone	And I hate my body because of these facts
Under the Arm	They are facts
Top of Head	They can't be changed

KEEP GOING TO
NEXT PAGE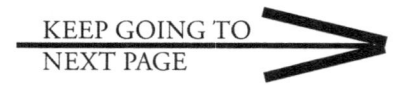

Eyebrow	I am stuck with this body
Side of Eye	And all of these faults
Under the Eye	I have a sluggish metabolism and I hate it
Nose	I am carb sensitive and I hate that too
Chin	I pack on fat quickly and I hate that about myself
Collarbone	I hate my body
Under the Arm	And I hate me
Top of Head	I can never be perfect enough to overcome all of this

 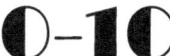 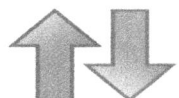

Eyebrow	That's what I have believed in the past
Side of Eye	But maybe it isn't all that true
Under the Eye	My metabolism is just energy and energy can change
Nose	Carb sensitivity is just energy and energy can change
Chin	Packing on fat is just a sign of how my energy is flowing
Collarbone	And that energy can change too
Under the Arm	I am open to the possibility that even these things can change
Top of Head	I choose to be awed and amazed at how my body can respond to loving thoughts and intentions

 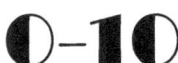 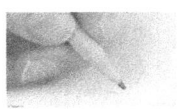

I am frustrated by my inability to control my eating.

The Setup

I am frustrated by my inability to control my eating. I like to control everything, and not being able to control myself is really scary. In spite of my frustration, and in spite of my lack of control, I choose to move forward with calm energy and confidence. Even though I am frustrated by my inability to control my eating, I deeply and completely love and respect my willingness to change this. I am relieved to know that I don't have to change this all at once, just one bite at a time.

The Tapping

Eyebrow	I am frustrated
Side of Eye	I don't feel like I can control my eating
Under the Eye	I am really bothered by this lack of control
Nose	I am frustrated
Chin	I can't ever seem to control my eating
Collarbone	Well, that's not completely true
Under the Arm	I can control my eating if it is something I don't like
Top of Head	That tells me I have some control

KEEP GOING TO NEXT PAGE

Eyebrow	I do like control
Side of Eye	I am frustrated whenever it looks like I am losing control
Under the Eye	In spite of this frustration I choose to remain calm
Nose	In spite of this frustration I choose to feel confident
Chin	I can learn to eat better one bite at a time
Collarbone	I am so glad to know that I don't have to change all at once
Under the Arm	I choose to focus on the times when I control my eating more easily
Top of Head	I am learning to be okay making small changes, one at a time

 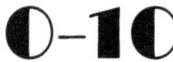 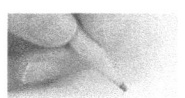

"Food is an important part of a balanced diet." - Fran Lebowitz

I hate vegetables.

The Setup

Even though I hate vegetables, I deeply and completely love and accept myself. Even though I think vegetables are totally disgusting, I love myself and my body anyway. I know I should eat vegetables, but I hate them. In spite of that, I choose to find ways to give my body the nourishment it really needs.

The Tapping

Eyebrow	I hate vegetables
Side of Eye	I hate to look at them
Under the Eye	I hate to cook them
Under the Nose	I hate to smell them
Chin	I hate to chop them
Collarbone	I hate to bite into them
Under the Arm	I hate to chew them
Top of Head	I hate vegetables

KEEP GOING TO NEXT PAGE

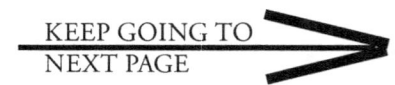

Eyebrow	They say vegetables are good for me
Side of Eye	But I hate them
Under the Eye	I want to be healthy
Nose	I don't really hate ALL vegetables
Chin	I just hate most of them
Collarbone	I am trying to eat better
Under the Arm	I hate some vegetables
Top of Head	I choose to be open to eating what my body needs, even if it means eating some vegetables

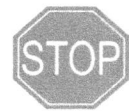 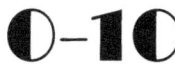 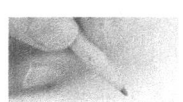

"Dieting is the only game where you win when you lose!" - Karl Lagerfeld

I feel hungry right now.

The Setup

I just ate, but I feel really hungry right now. I don't know why I feel hungry because it can't possibly be true. I already ate enough for this meal. I really want more though. Even though this feeling of hunger is very strong right now, I acknowledge that what I am feeling isn't really hunger. It is something else. This hunger feeling seems very real, but I choose to remember that I have just eaten. Even though I have these conflicting thoughts and feelings, I accept where I am right now.

The Tapping

Eyebrow	I feel hungry
Side of Eye	I want food right now
Under the Eye	I want this hunger feeling to go away
Nose	I feel hungry
Chin	All of my cells are crying out for food
Collarbone	No they're not
Under the Arm	Yes they are
Top of Head	No they're not

KEEP GOING TO
NEXT PAGE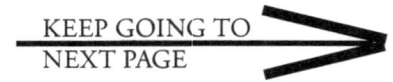

Eyebrow	It's not my body, it's my brain that wants food
Side of Eye	My dopamine receptors are confused
Under the Eye	My dopamine receptors in my brain are seeking pleasure, not food
Nose	Because that is true, I can do other pleasurable things to shut them up
Chin	It's up to me to un-confuse my brain
Collarbone	I don't have to listen to my dopamine receptors at this time
Under the Arm	I don't have to eat food right now
Top of Head	I can choose to use my frontal lobes instead

 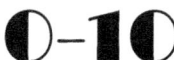 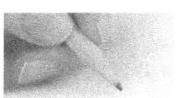

"People tend to be generous when sharing their nonsense, fear, and ignorance. And while they seem quite eager to feed you their negativity, please remember that sometimes the diet we need to be on is a spiritual and emotional one. Be cautious with what you feed your mind and soul. Fuel yourself with positivity and let that fuel propel you into positive action." - Steve Maraboli

I do not want to waste food.

The Setup

I was taught not to waste food. Everybody knows that it is wrong to waste food when there are starving people in other places. I was raised on that. Even though not cleaning my plate would be wasting food, I want to love and accept myself anyway. Wasting food is a big no no. I'm glad I'm doing my part to help the people that are starving by eating more food myself. That helps a lot. Even so, I choose to love and accept myself anyway. In spite of this current temptation to waste food, I choose to eat calmly and rationally.

The Tapping

Eyebrow	There is more food on my plate than my body needs
Side of Eye	There are starving people
Under the Eye	All over the world
Nose	So I have to eat ALL of the food
Chin	That will help them have food to eat
Collarbone	No it won't
Under the Arm	It won't help them at all if I eat this food
Top of Head	And it will actually hurt me

KEEP GOING TO NEXT PAGE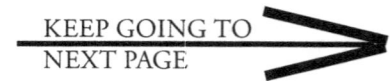

Eyebrow	In the future I can put less food on my plate
Side of Eye	Then I won't be tempted to overeat
Under the Eye	I can buy less food and send money to charity to feed the hungry
Nose	Then we can all be healthier
Chin	I can compost this extra food right now and help make better soil
Collarbone	When I eat less I can be healthier and do more to help others and myself
Under the Arm	It makes much more sense to eat less, spend less, and worry less
Top of Head	It makes sense to eat calmly and rationally

 **0-10**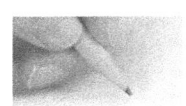

Tapping Exercise:

What happened when you exercised last? Think about when you exercised, what exercise you did, and how you felt. What were you wearing? What were you worried about while you were exercising? Tap about any negative thoughts or feelings surrounding your last exercise experience.

They will think I am rude if I do not eat it.

The Setup

I am afraid they will think I'm rude if I don't eat this food. Everybody else will be eating it. She'll probably think I am too picky or don't trust her cooking. They might even think I am a snob. I don't want people to think I am rude so I should just go ahead and eat. I accept how I am feeling right now and I love and accept me. I could try some of everything so that I can give honest feedback if I'm asked if I like it. I feel good about the part of me that wants to avoid being rude or inconsiderate.

The Tapping

Eyebrow	They will think I am rude if I do not eat it
Side of Eye	They might think I am too picky
Under the Eye	They might think I don't trust her cooking
Nose	What would I say if someone asks me if I liked something?
Chin	How would I explain myself?
Collarbone	Are these just excuses to indulge myself?
Under the Arm	Busted!
Top of Head	No one who really cares about me would want me to overeat or do something that is unhealthy

KEEP GOING TO NEXT PAGE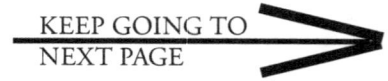

Eyebrow	I wouldn't have any trouble turning down tripe
Side of Eye	I wouldn't have any trouble turning down brussel sprouts
Under the Eye	That is probably a clue that this is just an excuse
Nose	I choose to consider other ways to handle the situation
Chin	I know lots of strategies for managing hunger
Collarbone	I know lots of strategies for managing impulse eating
Under the Arm	This isn't really about food anyway
Top of Head	People may actually be jealous of my self control. That would feel awesome

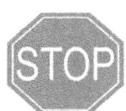 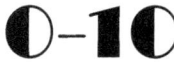 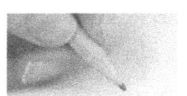

"Appetite has really become an artificial and abnormal thing, having taken the place of true hunger, which alone is natural. The one is a sign of bondage but the other, of freedom." - Paul Brunton

I am obese.

The Setup

I am obese. Those are hard words to say. Even though I really know that it is true, it feels very different to actually say it. Saying the words seems to make it even more real. All kinds of bad feelings come rushing in. Knowing that I am obese makes me feel pretty bad about myself. How can I possibly be happy knowing that I am obese. In spite of these feelings, I choose to love and accept myself even though my body isn't what I want it to be. Even though I don't know how to love and accept myself since I am obese, I choose to focus on all of the many loveable parts of me.

The Tapping

Eyebrow	I am obese
Side of Eye	I am obese
Under the Eye	I am obese
Nose	I am obese
Chin	I am obese
Collarbone	I am obese
Under the Arm	I am obese
Top of Head	I am obese

   **0-10**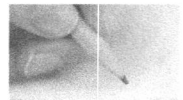

It's not fair that I'm fat and you're not.

The Setup

It's just not fair that I am far and you aren't. I hate saying that, but it is really how I feel. I know that my fat doesn't have anything to do with you, but it does feel like it. I choose to love myself, including my feelings. I choose to love myself, including my thoughts. I choose to love myself, and my insistence upon fairness.

The Tapping

Eyebrow	It doesn't feel fair that I'm fat
Side of Eye	Being fat just isn't fair
Under the Eye	It's not fair that I'm fat
Nose	And I'm looking for something to blame
Chin	I don't want to blame myself
Collarbone	So I'll just say its not fair
Under the Arm	Being fat just isn't fair
Top of Head	It doesn't feel fair that I'm fat

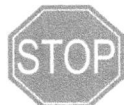 0–10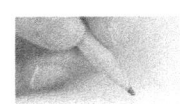

62

I'm as big as a house.

The Setup

I am as big as a house. That's not a very nice thing to say about myself, but it is true. Anyone who sees me would think that. In spite of being this big, I want to deeply and completely love and accept myself. Even though I am as big as a house, I am trying to have a more fit body. That is why I am tapping. Even though I am as big as a house, I am open to seeing myself as a work in progress.

The Tapping

Eyebrow	I am as big as a house
Side of Eye	That isn't a very nice expression
Under the Eye	It isn't even a very accurate expression
Nose	I am larger than I want to be
Chin	I am larger than is healthy for me
Collarbone	When I say I am as big as a house
Under the Arm	I am really exaggerating
Top of Head	I wonder why I need to tear myself down so much?

KEEP GOING TO NEXT PAGE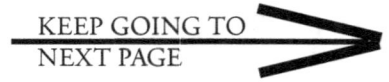

Eyebrow	Am I looking for sympathy?
Side of Eye	Maybe I want someone to say it isn't true
Under the Eye	Maybe I think it keeps me safe from having anybody else say bad things about me if I say it first
Nose	It is time to come up with a better metaphor
Chin	I'd be very small for a house
Collarbone	I'm even too small for an apartment
Under the Arm	I'm even too small to make a good tree house
Top of Head	The truth is, I'm just bigger than I want to be and I can change that

 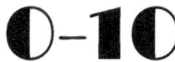 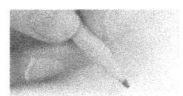

Tapping Exercise:

Start tapping. I want you to remember a time when someone criticized your appearance. Who made the criticism? How old were you? How did you react? Try to remember the exact words and situation. Keep tapping until your emotional reaction to this event is low. Are there more times when someone criticized the way you look? Tap on as many of them as you can remember.

I can't resist the chocolate chip cookies. They are my favorites.

The Setup

Even though I don't really think I can resist those chocolate chip cookies because they are my favorites, I love and accept myself anyway. I've never been able to resist chocolate chip cookies and I'm not sure I really want to resist them. If I eat them, I'll get even fatter than I already am. I want to love and accept myself, whether I eat the cookies or not.

The Tapping

Eyebrow	I don't think I can resist the chocolate chip cookies
Side of Eye	Those are my favorites
Under the Eye	I can't imagine not eating them right now
Nose	They really are my favorites
Chin	I love the way the chocolate chips melt in my mouth
Collarbone	I even like the dough before it is cooked
Under the Arm	I love the way they taste
Top of Head	I love the way they feel in my mouth

KEEP GOING TO NEXT PAGE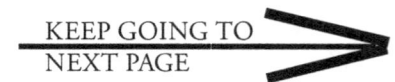

Eyebrow	I love the way they add inches to my hips when I eat them
Side of Eye	I love the way my jeans get tighter after just a dozen or so cookies
Under the Eye	What am I saying? No I don't
Nose	That's part of the problem
Chin	It probably wouldn't be so bad if I could stop at just one cookie
Collarbone	But I know myself better than that
Under the Arm	I've never stopped at just one chocolate chip cookie before
Top of Head	And I probably won't stop at just one now

 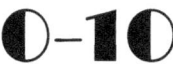 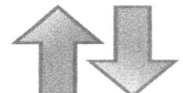

Eyebrow	It would be safer to not get started eating them
Side of Eye	It would probably be a good idea not to bake them
Under the Eye	It might be a good idea to let them just be a fond memory
Nose	It is true that they used to be my favorites
Chin	But getting thin and healthy is my new favorite
Collarbone	That's a lifetime of feeling good, not just a few cookies
Under the Arm	Sometimes that is hard to remember
Top of Head	But I'm worth the work it may take to change this pattern

 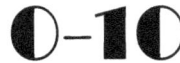 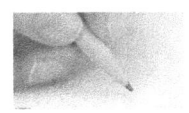

Dieting is getting really hard.

The Setup

This dieting is getting really hard. Anything that is this hard is probably too hard for me. Controlling my appetite is hard. Controlling my cravings is even harder than controlling my appetite. Planning ahead is hard. Avoiding sugary snacks is hard. Reading labels is hard. Eating a healthy diet is getting really hard. I don't want to do hard things. I want everything to be easy. I feel like giving up because this is hard. I acknowledge my frustration. I acknowledge my fatigue. I acknowledge my cravings. I acknowledge my appetite. I acknowledge my lack of energy and motivation. Most of all, I acknowledge that these feelings are okay and I'm okay.

The Tapping

Eyebrow	Dieting is really hard
Side of Eye	It's too hard for me
Under the Eye	I feel like giving up
Nose	I want to eat more food than my body needs
Chin	I don't want to plan ahead anymore
Collarbone	It's too much work
Under the Arm	It takes too much time
Top of Head	I want it to be easy

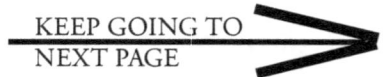

KEEP GOING TO
NEXT PAGE

Eyebrow	I am really frustrated right now
Side of Eye	I am frustrated with my body
Under the Eye	I am frustrated with my metabolism
Nose	I am so tired of this
Chin	This dieting is very hard
Collarbone	I am losing my motivation
Under the Arm	This dieting is getting really hard
Top of Head	It's just too hard

 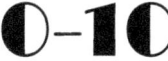 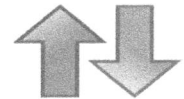

Eyebrow	I don't like these feelings
Side of Eye	I don't believe I should really feel this way
Under the Eye	I'm supposed to enjoy everything all the time
Nose	There must be something wrong with me
Chin	I am trying
Collarbone	I haven't given up yet
Under the Arm	These feelings are only temporary
Top of Head	It may be hard, but I choose to remember that I am worth it

 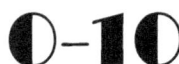 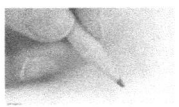

Food makes me happy.

The Setup

Even though food makes me happy, and eating food also makes me sad, and eating food also makes me angry, I deeply and completely love and accept myself and these conflicting emotions. Even though eating food makes me happy, I choose to look for other ways to make myself happy too. Even though eating food makes me sad, I choose to eat foods that nourish my body and my soul. Even though eating food often results in feeling angry with myself because I ate too much of the "wrong" things, I am learning to love and accept myself and my body anyway.

The Tapping

Eyebrow	Food makes me happy
Side of Eye	Food makes me happy
Under the Eye	I want to be happy so I have to eat
Nose	When I feel sad, I have to eat so I can be happy
Chin	When I am angry, I have to eat so I can be happy
Collarbone	When I am afraid, I have to eat so I can be happy
Under the Arm	Food is the only thing in my life that could possibly make me happy
Top of Head	Being with my family can't make me happy

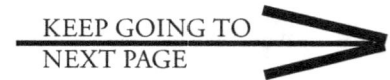

KEEP GOING TO
NEXT PAGE

Eyebrow	Spending time with friends could never make me happy
Side of Eye	Getting kissed by my dog couldn't make me happy
Under the Eye	Hiking, meditation, a warm bath, music, dancing, or taking a nap could never make me happy
Chin	That's ridiculous
Collarbone	Many things could add to my happiness if I let them
Under the Arm	I could choose to feel happier right now if I wanted to
Top of Head	I can do that with or without food

 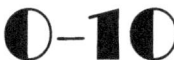 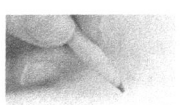

Tapping Exercise:

What is the first thought that pops in your mind when you think about exercise? Write it down, then spend some time tapping about it.

It doesn't feel like Thanksgiving without the pumpkin pie.

The Setup

It's Thanksgiving Day and there is food everywhere. What I like best is the pumpkin pie with whipped cream. It just doesn't feel like Thanksgiving if I don't eat the pumpkin pie. I want a great big piece just smothered with whipped cream. It tastes really good. It also makes me feel good. Even though I have these strong feelings about pumpkin pie, I deeply and completely love and accept myself.

The Tapping

Eyebrow	I want the pumpkin pie
Side of Eye	I want the pumpkin pie with whipped cream
Under the Eye	It wouldn't feel like Thanksgiving without the pumpkin pie
Nose	Where did I learn that Thanksgiving is all about the food?
Chin	When I first learned about Thanksgiving in school no one even mentioned pumpkin pie
Collarbone	What I learned about was mostly vegetables
Under the Arm	Why am I not craving the vegetables as a symbol for Thanksgiving?
Top of Head	I seem to have this all mixed up in my head

KEEP GOING TO NEXT PAGE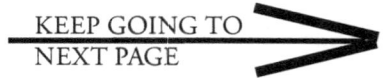

Eyebrow	I guess it's time to unmix it
Side of Eye	Part of me knows that pumpkin pie is just another dessert and doesn't really have any special power
Under the Eye	I could choose to focus on other aspects of Thanksgiving
Nose	I could choose to focus on the people and relationships
Chin	That would feel like Thanksgiving
Collarbone	I could choose to focus on gratitude
Under the Arm	That would make it feel like Thanksgiving
Top of Head	I am glad that there are other things to focus on during this holiday. Abstaining from pumpkin pie won't really ruin the day

 **0-10**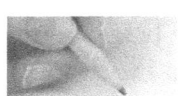

"Any food that requires enhancing by the use of chemical substances should in no way be considered a food." - John H. Tobe

I hate the treadmill.

The Setup

I really hate the treadmill. I just can't seem to make myself do it. It seems awful to walk without getting anywhere. Even though I really hate the treadmill and I rarely do any cardio workout, I choose to love and accept myself anyway. Even though I have definitely neglected my cardio workouts, I deeply and completely love and accept that part of myself that is at least trying to do what my body needs. Even though I really hate walking on the treadmill, I choose to be amazed by how easy it could seem in the future.

The Tapping

Eyebrow	I hate walking on the treadmill
Side of Eye	I really hate doing cardio
Under the Eye	It is just so boring
Nose	I know that doing more cardio would be a good thing
Chin	I know that walking on the treadmill and doing other cardio would help me lose even more weight
Collarbone	But I have been unable to make myself do it in the past
Under the Arm	What if there is a way to actually feel good about doing it?
Top of Head	What if it doesn't have to be awful?

KEEP GOING TO
NEXT PAGE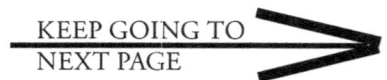

Eyebrow	I could focus on how good it feels to take care of myself
Side of Eye	I could focus on how my overall fitness
Under the Eye	Has improved as I am faithful to my workouts
Nose	I could use my cardio time to acknowledge
Chin	Everything thatI have to be grateful for
Collarbone	I could use my treadmill time to send positive energy to situations and people that are important to me
Under the Arm	I am starting to feel a little bit more positive about walking on the treadmill.
Top of Head	I am starting to feel a little bit more confident in my ability to do a regular cardio routine

   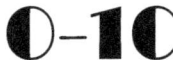   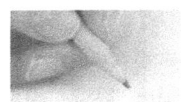

Tapping Exercise:

Was there ever a time when you experienced real hunger? If so, start tapping and remember the experience in as much detail as you can.

My whole family is overweight.

Setup

My whole family is overweight. I think I am genetically screwed. This situation feels pretty hopeless. Even though I feel helpless to address my weight issues since all of my relatives are overweight, I love and accept myself anyway. I choose to be awed and amazed at how easy it will be for me to reach a healthy weight, even though it would be easy to blame my weight on my faulty genes. Even though my ancestors may have been overweight, that doesn't necessarily mean that I have to be. I choose to do the things that I can do to get and stay healthy.

Tapping

Eyebrow	I have bad genes
Side of Eye	And my family has always been overweight
Under the Eye	I've always been overweight
Nose	I'm predestined to be overweight
Chin	There is nothing I can do to overcome that
Collarbone	I know that isn't really true
Under the Arm	But it feels true
Top of Head	Science tells me that there is a lot I can do about my weight

KEEP GOING TO NEXT PAGE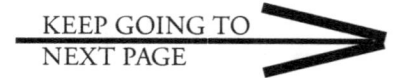

Eyebrow	It might be more difficult for me than people with thin genes
Side of Eye	But it might not be more difficult
Under the Eye	History doesn't determine the future
Nose	And my family's weight problem doesn't necessarily determine mine
Chin	Even though I believe that my genes may make weight loss more difficult for me
Collarbone	I choose to allow my weight loss to be easy
Under the Arm	I choose to allow my weight loss to be almost effortless
Top of Head	I choose to take control of my own future

 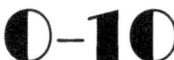 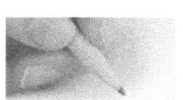

"Food, like your money, should be working for you!" - Rita Deattrea Beckford, M.D.

I don't think rationally about food.

The Setup

Even though I have trouble thinking rationally about food, I choose to love myself anyway. Even though I have trouble thinking rationally about food, I choose to accept my feelings anyway. Even though I have trouble thinking rationally about food, I choose to accept my thoughts about this anyway.

The Tapping

Eyebrow	I'm not very rational about food
Side of Eye	I'm not very rational about food
Under the Eye	I'm not very rational about food
Nose	I'm not very rational about food
Chin	I'm not very rational about food
Collarbone	I'm not very rational about food
Under the Arm	I'm not very rational about food
Top of Head	I'm not very rational about food

   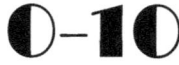   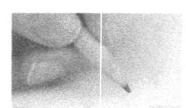

It feels like food is my only friend.

The Setup

Even though it feels like food is my only friend, I am open to learning to love myself anyway. I know it isn't really true that food is my only friend, but people sometimes disappoint me. It feels like food is my only friend, because food seems so much more reliable than people. Even though it feels like food is my only friend, I choose to handle my disappointments in other ways. Even though people sometimes let me down, I choose to let food remain food and friends remain friends.

Tapping

Eyebrow	Food is my only friend
Side of Eye	Food is my only friend
Under the Eye	Food is my only friend
Nose	Food is my only friend
Chin	Food is my only friend
Collarbone	Food is my only friend
Under the Arm	Food is my only friend
Top of Head	Food is my only friend

   **0-10**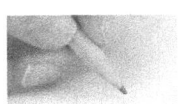

Eating healthy is too expensive.

The Setup

Even though I believe that eating healthy is too expensive and I can't afford it, I deeply and completely love and accept myself anyway. Even though eating healthy is too expensive for me, I honor that part of me that is doing the best I can. Even though I believe that eating healthy is just too expensive right now, I love and accept myself anyway. Healthy food is too expensive. The high carb stuff is much more affordable. I love and accept myself anyway.

The Tapping

Eyebrow	Healthy food is too expensive
Side of Eye	The high carb stuff is much more affordable
Under the Eye	I know I should be more careful about my diet
Nose	Sometimes I really try
Chin	But then someone will offer me a meal or something to eat
Collarbone	And it would be crazy to refuse a free meal
Under the Arm	These people are just being nice
Top of Head	And I really could use the help

KEEP GOING TO NEXT PAGE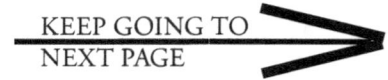

Eyebrow	Beggars can't be choosers
Side of Eye	And these meals aren't always the most healthy meals I've ever seen
Under the Eye	Sometimes they are deep fried
Nose	And there's almost always a great dessert
Chin	How can I turn that down?
Collarbone	I guess I could watch out for my portion size
Under the Arm	And I don't have to take a second portion
Top of Head	I could eat the portion that is right for my body

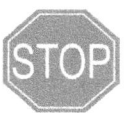 **0-10**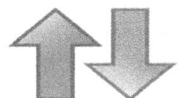

Eyebrow	I could even skip the dessert altogether
Side of Eye	Or ask if I could take it with me and eat it tomorrow when there isn't as much food
Under the Eye	I do have some choices I guess
Nose	I am not really helpless here
Chin	An apple isn't really any more expensive than some of the junk food I buy
Collarbone	Some healthy foods are more expensive than junk foods
Under the Arm	But if I pay attention, I can still take care of my body on a low budget
Top of Head	It feels good to know I have choices

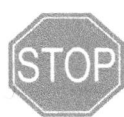 **0-10**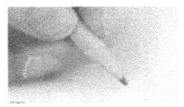

Other people sabotage my eating.

The Setup

Even though other people always sabotage me when I am trying to eat healthy, I love and accept myself anyway. Even though I can't diet because other people sabotage me, I love and accept myself and my attempts to eat better. Even though I keep letting other people sabotage me when I try to eat better, I choose to stick to my eating plan as much as possible.

The Tapping

Eyebrow	Whenever I try to diet
Side of Eye	Other people always sabotage me
Under the Eye	They may be doing it on purpose
Nose	Or they may be doing it accidentally
Chin	Either way, the result is the same
Collarbone	I don't reach my goals
Under the Arm	It is just too hard to stick to the plan when other people offer me those forbidden foods
Top of Head	Then there are those donuts at work

KEEP GOING TO NEXT PAGE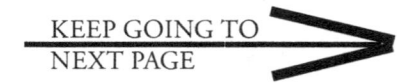

Eyebrow	Whenever I decide to diet, there seems to be food everywhere
Side of Eye	I can't resist that
Under the Eye	I want other people to stop sabotaging me
Nose	I want me to stop sabotaging myself
Chin	I want to be more in control of my choices
Collarbone	I choose to eat foods that make me happy and healthy
Under the Arm	Letting the behavior of other people get in my way isn't very smart
Top of Head	I choose to eat my way

 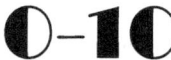 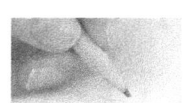

"Positive energy is your priceless life force.
Protect it." - Charlene Johnson

I need a quick pick me up.

The Setup

I'm really dragging and I need a quick pick me up. Food always works for that. It doesn't really fit with my diet, but I don't know what else to do. I don't have time for a nap and I need to get going fast. Even though I feel like I need a quick pick me up, I choose to remember that I have choices. Even though food always works to pick me up, that doesn't mean other things won't work for me too. I choose to keep my options open and make good long-term decisions. Even though I'm really dragging right now, I deeply and completely love and accept myself.

The Tapping

Eyebrow	I need a quick pick me up
Side of Eye	I'm really dragging right now
Under the Eye	I don't know what else to do since food always works
Nose	I don't really want to over eat
Chin	The things I want to eat aren't on my food plan
Collarbone	I've got to get things done
Under the Arm	And I need to get going now
Top of Head	Food always works

KEEP GOING TO NEXT PAGE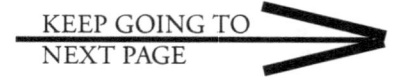

Eyebrow	Can I really pass up a sure thing?
Side of Eye	I need a pick me up now
Under the Eye	I guess I could try a few other things
Nose	A quick walk might work
Chin	Meditation might work too
Collarbone	Calling a good friend and laughing always feels good
Under the Arm	I don't feel good for very long when I overeat
Top of Head	Blowing my diet always makes me mad at myself too. I'm really glad I took the time to think this through. I feel better already

 **0–10**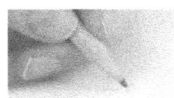

Tapping Exercise:

Where does your energy go? Many of us use food as a pick me up, but what are we picking ourselves up from? Finish this statement, "It seems like my energy is going ...." Now visualize the process of your energy leaving you. Tap about any thoughts or feelings that arise.

I can't lose weight because I don't like to exercise.

The Setup

Even though I can't lose weight because I don't like to exercise, I love and accept myself completely. Even though I can't lose weight because I don't like to exercise, I love and accept myself completely. Even though I can't lose weight because I don't like to exercise, I love and accept myself completely.

The Tapping

Eyebrow	I can't lose weight
Side of Eye	Because I don't like to exercise
Under the Eye	I certainly can't do it just by diet alone
Nose	So I might as well give up
Chin	I hate to exercise
Collarbone	It doesn't feel good
Under the Arm	I get all out of breath
Top of Head	I sweat

KEEP GOING TO NEXT PAGE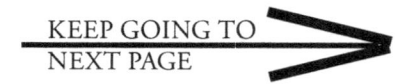

Eyebrow	And its really hard
Side of Eye	People that like it must be crazy
Under the Eye	Since I don't like to exercise I can't lose weight
Nose	I just can't lose weight
Chin	I don't like to exercise
Collarbone	I don't even really like to move
Under the Arm	I could just sit in one place forever and never exercise at all
Top of Head	I never walk

 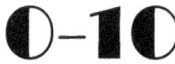 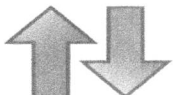

Eyebrow	I never do chores
Side of Eye	I never go shopping
Under the Eye	I never play
Nose	I never dance
Chin	I never do anything that involves movement
Collarbone	Well, that's not true
Under the Arm	I do move, and I guess that really is exercise
Top of Head	I am open to learning how to move more and eat less. It's good to know that I don't have to do it all at once

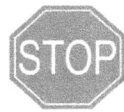 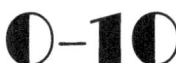 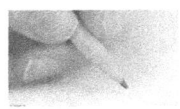

I just can't resist that Halloween candy.

The Setup

Even though I don't believe that I can resist that Halloween candy, I accept myself, knowing that I have this limitation. Even though I've never been able to resist that Halloween candy, I love knowing that I can choose not to have it around me at all if I don't want to. Even though I can't resist that Halloween candy, I choose to make rational decisions about buying it, eating it, and giving it away.

The Tapping

Eyebrow	I can't resist that Halloween candy
Side of Eye	I start eating it almost as soon as I buy it
Under the Eye	Then if there is any left I have to eat it
Nose	I couldn't let it go to waste
Chin	Those candies are so small that they don't seem like they should be a problem
Collarbone	But I never stop with just one
Under the Arm	I've finished a whole bag of candy before Trick or Treat night even starts
Top of Head	I hate that feeling of being out of control

KEEP GOING TO NEXT PAGE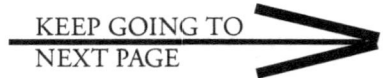

Eyebrow	Part of me believes it doesn't have to be that way
Side of Eye	But I've never been successful before
Under the Eye	I just don't think I can resist
Nose	I choose to honor my conflict
Chin	I know I will feel bad about my lack of control if I eat it
Collarbone	But I will feel good for those few minutes when I am eating the candy
Under the Arm	Eating as much candy as I want makes me feel like a kid again
Top of Head	I choose to love and accept myself no matter what I decide

 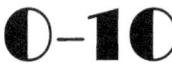 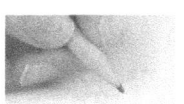

"I finally figured out the big, elusive secret to weight loss. Don't eat! Who knew?" - Richelle E. Goodrich

I just ate 3 brownies. I am such a failure.

The Setup

Even though I just ate 3 brownies, and they definitely weren't on my food plan for this afternoon, I choose to love and accept myself anyway. Even though I ate 3 brownies while waiting for my lunch to cook, I choose to love and accept myself anyway. Even though I feel like a failure since I ate those brownies, I choose to love and accept myself anyway.

The Tapping

Eyebrow	I just ate 3 brownies
Side of Eye	I can't believe it
Under the Eye	I had been doing so well
Nose	This seems like a huge setback
Chin	It's not like I was really hungry
Collarbone	I am actually cooking lunch right now
Under the Arm	I am nervous that it won't be good
Top of Head	I've made two dishes that I've never made before

KEEP GOING TO NEXT PAGE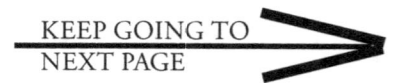

Eyebrow	That always makes me anxious
Side of Eye	But I'm also excited to see what happens
Under the Eye	I know that I often eat when I am nervous
Nose	Next time I may want to plan for a healthy snack while my new recipes are cooking
Chin	Getting off of my food plan with these brownies isn't a total disaster, just a setback
Collarbone	I can get back on track right now
Under the Arm	In fact, I AM back on track right now
Top of Head	I feel better already

   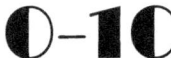   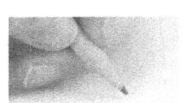

"A dark chocolate truffle melts in my mouth, and I forget about everything else...even the fact that I'm on a diet." - Barbara Brooke

Wine helps me relax in the evening.

The Setup

Even though wine helps me relax in the evening, I know that it adds to the calories I'm taking in each day. I don't even want to think about giving that up too. I've already given up so many foods that I love in order to lose weight. Giving up my wine just doesn't feel like it is even possible. What would I do to relax in the evenings instead? Even though this conflict feels very uncomfortable to me, I am open to wisdom and clarity. Even though I am reluctant to give up my glass of wine in the evening, and I suspect that it is making it harder for me to reach my weight loss goals, I love and accept myself anyway.

The Tapping

Eyebrow	Wine helps me relax in the evening
Side of Eye	I just don't know what I would do without it
Under the Eye	I am afraid that I would be uptight and anxious
Nose	I certainly don't want that
Chin	Besides, they say wine is good for you
Collarbone	It's almost a health food
Under the Arm	I really do know better than that
Top of Head	I don't like the idea that I have to drink wine just to relax

KEEP GOING TO NEXT PAGE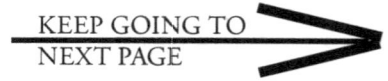

Eyebrow	It would be nice if I could come up with some other things that relax me too
Side of Eye	Maybe things that don't have so many calories
Under the Eye	Or even things that burn calories
Nose	That would be nice
Chin	I could ask for help so I don't feel overwhelmed
Collarbone	Wine does help me relax in the evening
Under the Arm	Adding all of those calories on to the end of my day isn't really what I want in the long run
Top of Head	But I don't want anybody to take it away from me

 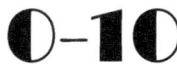 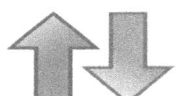

Eyebrow	I am choosing what calories I want to put in my body
Side of Eye	Sometimes I might plan my day so that I have a glass of wine
Under the Eye	Some days I might not
Nose	Nothing bad will happen to me if I don't drink the wine
Chin	There are lots of ways I can take care of myself
Collarbone	It feels good to know that I have choices
Under the Arm	It feels good to take care of myself
Top of Head	It feels good to know I can always tap if I need to relax

 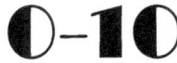 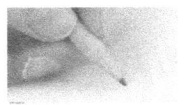

78

I just can't do it anymore.

The Setup

Dieting is just too hard. I don't feel like I can do it any more. I really want it to be easier. I am so tired of this Even though dieting feels too hard right now, I choose to remember how strong I really am. Even though dieting feels too hard right now, I choose to remember how capable I really am. Even though it feels like I just can't do it anymore, I choose to love and accept myself anyway.

The Tapping

Eyebrow	Dieting is too hard
Side of Eye	I just can't do it anymore
Under the Eye	Dieting is too hard
Nose	I just can't do it anymore
Chin	Dieting is too hard
Collarbone	I just can't do it anymore
Under the Arm	Dieting is too hard
Top of Head	I just can't do it anymore

   0-10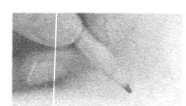

I have so many excuses.

The Setup

Even though I have so many excuses about why I can't lose weight, I love and accept myself and all of my feelings anyway. Even though I have so many excuses about why I can't lose weight, I love and accept myself and all of my thoughts anyway. Even though I have so many excuses about why I can't lose weight, I love and accept myself and all of my many excuses too.

The Tapping

Eyebrow	So many excuses
Side of Eye	I have all of these excuses
Under the Eye	These excuses
Nose	So many excuses
Chin	I have so many excuses
Collarbone	All of these excuses
Under the Arm	These excuses
Top of Head	So many excuses

   **0-10**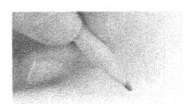

80

I feel overwhelmed by how far I still have to go.

The Setup

I'm feeling overwhelmed. I've lost weight, but I still have a long way to go before I reach my weight loss goal. Sometimes I feel like giving up. I've come a long way, but I feel overwhelmed when I think about continuing on to my goal. Even though I am feeling overwhelmed, I choose to remember how good it feels to be losing weight. Even though I am feeling overwhelmed, I choose to allow my future weight loss to be much easier than it has been in the past.

The Tapping

Eyebrow	I'm feeling overwhelmed
Side of Eye	Feeling overwhelmed
Under the Eye	I have so far to go
Nose	This feeling of being overwhelmed
Chin	I'm overwhelmed
Collarbone	I have a long way to go
Under the Eye	I am so overwhelmed
Top of Head	My goal seems so far away

KEEP GOING TO NEXT PAGE
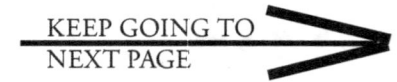

Eyebrow	I am feeling overwhelmed
Side of Eye	But I choose to remember the feeling of success
Under the Eye	I am feeling overwhelmed
Nose	But I choose to allow weight loss to get easier and easier
Chin	I am feeling overwhelmed
Collarbone	But I choose to feel relaxed and calm
Under the Arm	I am feeling overwhelmed
Top of Head	But I choose to feel successful and confident

 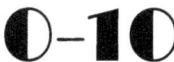 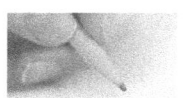

"Successful people do what others know they should do but will not. To become a success, or just be *more* successful, you will do what average, less-motivated people will not." - Charlene Johnson

I can't wear the clothes that are in my closet.

The Setup

Even though I feel frustrated that I can't wear the clothes that are in my closet, I love and accept myself anyway. Even though I feel frustrated that I can't wear the clothes that are in my closet, I love and accept myself anyway. Even though I feel frustrated that I can't wear the clothes that are in my closet, I love and accept myself anyway.

The Tapping

Eyebrow	This frustration
Side of Eye	This frustration
Under the Eye	All of this frustration
Nose	This frustration about my clothes
Chin	I can't wear most of them
Collarbone	Because I have gained weight
Under the Arm	I am so frustrated
Top of Head	I have lots of clothes in my closet

KEEP GOING TO NEXT PAGE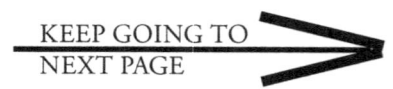

Eyebrow	I can't wear them
Side of Eye	That is so frustrating
Under the Eye	All of this clothing frustration
Nose	I am so frustrated
Chin	All of those clothes in my closet
Collarbone	And they don't fit
Under the Arm	This clothing frustration
Top of Head	All of this clothing frustration

 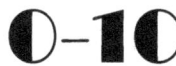 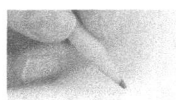

Tapping Exercise:

Look at your arms. Do you see muscles? Are they flabby or floppy? Do they look strong? How do you feel when you look at your arms? What are the first words that pop into your head? Start tapping.

I am embarrassed to be seen in public.

The Setup

Even though I am embarrassed to be seen in public, I am open to learning better ways to cope. Even though I am embarrassed to be seen in public, I am open to feeling more comfortable in the future. Even though I am embarrassed to be seen in public, I am willing to love and accept myself anyway.

The Tapping

Eyebrow	I am embarrassed to be seen in public
Side of Eye	I feel like everyone is looking at me
Under the Eye	I feel like everyone is judging me
Nose	And why not?
Chin	I am judging me
Collarbone	I feel like my body is hideous
Under the Arm	I look ugly
Top of Head	I look fat

KEEP GOING TO NEXT PAGE
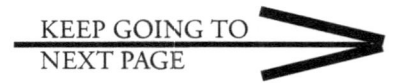

Eyebrow	My clothes don't fit properly
Side of Eye	I can only imagine what other people think
Under the Eye	But if it is as bad as what I think
Nose	It is really terrible
Chin	I am embarrassed to be seen in public
Collarbone	I don't want to be looked at
Under the Arm	I don't want to be judged
Top of Head	Not by other people and not by me

 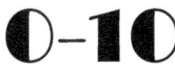 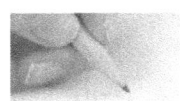

"If you do just one thing - make one conscious choice - that can change the world, go organic." - Maria Rodale

I want Valentine's Day candy.

The Setup

It seems wrong to celebrate Valentine's Day without candy. I've always given and received candy for Valentine's Day. I really like the chocolates, but I even like the little candy hearts. Neither one is healthy. Neither is part of my food plan. That makes me feel sad. I know the candy isn't really what the holiday is about, but it feels like something will be missing. Even though I have all of these conflicted feelings and thoughts about Valentine's Day candy, I deeply and completely love and accept myself. Even though I feel conflicted about Valentine's Day candy, I choose to embrace the conflict. Even though I feel sad about giving up Valentine's Day candy, I acknowledge my feelings. I acknowledge my thoughts. I love and accept myself anyway.

The Tapping

Eyebrow	I want Valentine's Day candy
Side of Eye	I want Valentine's Day candy
Under the Eye	I want Valentine's Day candy
Nose	I want Valentine's Day candy
Chin	I want Valentine's Day candy
Collarbone	I want Valentine's Day candy
Under the Arm	I want Valentine's Day candy
Top of Head	I want the chocolate

KEEP GOING TO NEXT PAGE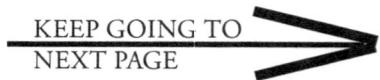

Eyebrow	I want the candy hearts
Side of Eye	I want Valentine's Day candy
Under the Eye	I want chocolate
Nose	I want candy hearts
Chin	I want it all
Collarbone	I want Valentine's Day candy
Under the Arm	I really want it
Top of Head	I want Valentine's Day candy

 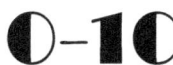 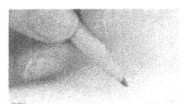

Tapping Exercise:

What comments have you heard about your food choices? Start tapping and recall as many of the comments as you can. Try to remember who made the comment, what they were commenting about, who overheard the comment, and your responses.

I was stuffing food in my mouth.

The Setup

I was just stuffing food in my mouth. I was barely finishing one cookie before I started the other one. I didn't even taste them after a while. Why would I do that to myself? I know I was upset. I know I was frustrated. I know I felt hurt and angry. My head tells me that it isn't a good enough reason to eat like that because it won't really help. Being that out of control is scary for me. Even though I am disgusted by my eating, I acknowledge all of the emotions that contributed to my behavior. Even though I am upset about my senseless eating, I acknowledge my thoughts and feelings. Even though I hate being that out of control of my emotions and my eating, I would like to learn to love and accept myself more completely.

The Tapping

Eyebrow	I was stuffing food in my mouth
Side of Eye	I was really out of control
Under the Eye	I am not happy about that
Nose	I was angry
Chin	So I stuffed food in my mouth
Collarbone	I was upset
Under the Arm	So I stuffed food in my mouth
Top of Head	I was frustrated

KEEP GOING TO NEXT PAGE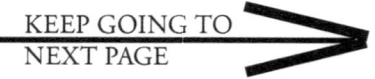

Eyebrow	So I stuffed food in my mouth
Side of Eye	I felt hurt
Under the Eye	So I stuffed food in my mouth
Nose	I am so disgusted by my behavior
Chin	I know that stuffing food in my mouth won't really solve any of my problems
Collarbone	It didn't really make me feel better either
Under the Arm	I was just stuffing food in my mouth
Top of Head	That is embarrassing

 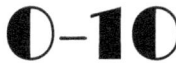 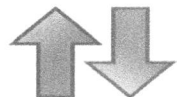

Eyebrow	Even though I was stuffing food in my mouth
Side of Eye	I choose to learn other ways to handle my mood
Under the Eye	Even though I was stuffing food in my mouth
Nose	I am open to learning more about my feelings
Chin	Even though I was just stuffing food in my mouth
Collarbone	I choose to address my feelings in a more healthy manner
Under the Arm	Even though I was just stuffing food in my mouth
Top of Head	I choose to consider my options before I eat

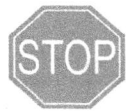 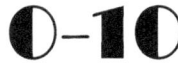 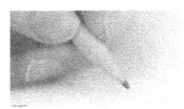

I must do this perfectly.

The Setup

It's hard to even get started because I feel like I must do this perfectly. That makes it hard to diet. It makes it hard to exercise. It makes it hard to do anything to even begin to lose the weight. In spite of this difficulty, I am open to learning to think about things differently. In spite of these challenges, I am open to a change in the way I feel about things. In spite of this, I am open to learning to love and accept myself and all of my imperfections.

The Tapping

Eyebrow	I feel like I must do this perfectly
Side of Eye	And that makes it really hard to get started
Under the Eye	I feel like I must do everything perfectly
Nose	And that usually gets me nowhere
Chin	I am ready to try something new
Collarbone	But it feels almost impossible
Under the Arm	I am open to learning to love and accept myself anyway
Top of Head	I feel like I have to do this perfectly

KEEP GOING TO NEXT PAGE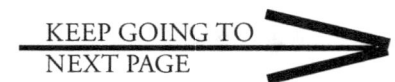

Eyebrow	I am open to guidance and clarity
Side of Eye	This perfection thing is bothersome
Under the Eye	I choose not to let my need for perfection get in the way of my goals and dreams
Nose	I would like to do things perfectly
Chin	But I accept that sometimes it may not be possible
Collarbone	I don't want to fail
Under the Arm	But sometimes I could measure success a little differently
Top of Head	I am open to guidance and clarity

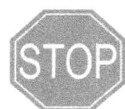 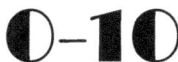 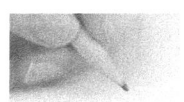

"Nothing in the world can take the place of persistence.
Talent will not; nothing is more common than unsuccessful
men with talent. Genius will not; unrewarded genius is almost
a proverb. Education will not; the world is full of educated
derelicts. Persistence and determination alone are omnipotent.
The slogan Press On! has solved and always will solve the
problems of the human race." - J. Calvin Coolidge

I am afraid that I will choose the wrong plan.

The Setup

Even though I am afraid I will choose the wrong diet plan, I am willing to face my fear and take meaningful action. Even though I am afraid that I will choose the wrong diet plan, I acknowledge that doing something has got to be better than doing nothing. Even though I am afraid that I will choose the wrong diet plan, I love and accept myself anyway.

The Tapping

Eyebrow	I am afraid that I will choose the wrong diet plan
Side of Eye	I know that fear is the wrong motivation for most decision making
Under the Eye	I am afraid I will choose the wrong diet plan
Nose	There is so much conflicting information out there
Chin	What if I choose the wrong one?
Collarbone	That thought makes me nervous
Under the Arm	I would like to listen to my body
Top of Head	And learn what it needs to be healthy

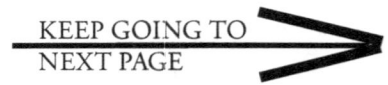

KEEP GOING TO NEXT PAGE

Eyebrow	I want clarity about this decision
Side of Eye	I don't want to feel afraid about this anymore
Under the Eye	I want to move forward toward health with calm confidence
Nose	Even though I have been afraid that I might choose the wrong diet plan
Chin	I am open to feeling surprisingly calm about making this decision
Collarbone	I have had all of this fear
Under the Arm	And it has been holding me back
Top of Head	But it won't hold me back any more

 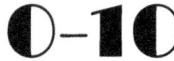 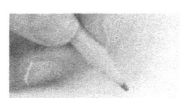

Tapping Exercise:

While tapping through the points, describe your biggest diet failure.

I am afraid that the diet will not work for me.

The Setup

Even though I am afraid that the diet won't work for me, I am open to seeing this in a new way. Even though I'm afraid that the diet won't work for me, I am open to seeing this in a new way. I choose to love and accept myself anyway. Even though I am afraid that the diet won't work for me, I choose to believe that I can get through this uncertainty.

The Tapping

Eyebrow	I am afraid that the diet will not work for me
Side of Eye	I have all of this fear
Under the Eye	What if it doesn't work?
Nose	Will I be any worse than I am right now?
Chin	I am afraid that the diet will not work for me
Collarbone	I have this paralyzing fear
Under the Arm	I am afraid that the diet will not work for me
Top of Head	I am afraid that the diet will not work for me

   **0–10**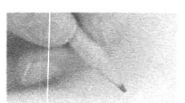

I'm mad at myself for failing again.

The Setup

I am so incredibly mad at myself for failing again. I keep saying that I'm going to stick to my eating plan, but I didn't. I failed. Even though I feel like I've failed again, I choose to love the person inside. I acknowledge that I am feeling mad at myself and I choose to accept that feeling. Even though I'm mad at myself for failing again, I love and accept myself in spite of this frustration.

The Tapping

Eyebrow	I'm mad at myself
Side of Eye	I'm feeling really mad at myself right now
Under the Eye	I feel like I've let myself down
Nose	I'm mad at myself for failing to follow my own food plan
Chin	I am so mad at myself right now
Collarbone	It makes sense to be mad right now
Under the Arm	I'm so mad at myself
Top of Head	I hate failing at anything, but particularly this

0-10

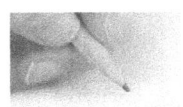

I'm upset so I eat.

The Setup

Even though I eat when I am upset, I love and accept myself anyway. Even though I eat whenever I am upset, I love and accept myself anyway. I eat when I am upset. I love and accept myself anyway, in spite of this behavior that I see as a flaw.

The Tapping

Eyebrow	When I am upset I eat
Side of Eye	When I am upset I eat
Under the Eye	When I am upset I feel compelled to eat
Nose	I'm not sure that is really true
Chin	When I am upset I've developed a habit of eating
Collarbone	That feels more true to me
Under the Arm	When I am upset I have a habit of eating that I would like to change
Top of Head	When I am upset I have a habit of eating

KEEP GOING TO NEXT PAGE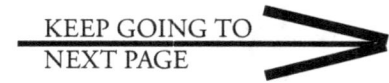

Eyebrow	And I would like to change that
Side of Eye	When I am upset I eat
Under the Eye	But it doesn't have to be that way because it is just a habit
Nose	Habits can change
Chin	That means I can respond in another way when I am upset
Collarbone	It is not realistic to expect that I'll never be upset
Under the Arm	It's not realistic to expect that I won't eat
Top of Head	But they do not have to go together

 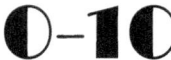 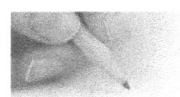

"Find something to feel good about and get out of the way, and allow the cells to receive what they've been asking for. That is the key to healing." - Abraham Hicks

One brownie just isn't enough.

The Setup

Even though one brownie just isn't enough, I love and accept myself anyway. Even though I always want more than just one brownie, I love and accept myself and my appetite for sweets. Even though I always want more when I eat a brownie, I love and accept myself completely.

The Tapping

Eyebrow	I love brownies
Side of Eye	I love brownies and all kinds of sweets
Under the Eye	Eating just one doesn't seem like a real option for me
Nose	If I eat one, I always want two, or three, or four
Chin	It's almost impossible to stop after one
Collarbone	I get frustrated that I don't seem to have any self control
Under the Arm	My brain knows that one brownie should be enough
Top of Head	Eating more than one doesn't really make me feel any better

KEEP GOING TO NEXT PAGE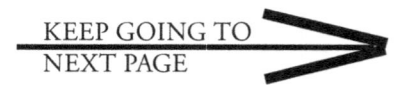

Eyebrow	Eating more does seem to prolong the time I get to experience the pleasure
Side of Eye	Maybe if I could slow down I could enjoy the pleasure for a longer time without overeating
Under the Eye	That's what I really want
Nose	I want to feel good for a longer period of time
Chin	I am open to other ways to feel pleasure
Collarbone	I can feel pleasure without eating more food than is healthy for my body
Under the Arm	I can enjoy one brownie
Top of Head	I am excited to think I could even enjoy just half a brownie someday

 **0–10**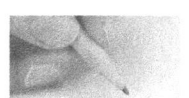

"Life is a tragedy of nutrition." - Arnold Ehret

Potato Chips

The Setup

Tonight my problem was potato chips. At least they weren't regular potato chips. These were actually fancy vegetable chips. While I'd like to feel better about that, the truth is that I still ate too much. I ate too many calories. I ate too late at night. I wish I had more control over my eating. I wish I had more control over my snacking. Tonight my problem was potato chips. In spite of all of this, I choose to love and accept myself anyway.

The Tapping

Eyebrow	I ate potato chips tonight
Side of Eye	I didn't measure them
Under the Eye	I ate too many of them
Nose	That makes me feel bad
Chin	Physically and mentally
Collarbone	I wish I had more control over my eating
Under the Arm	Really, I wish I didn't need to control my eating at all
Top of Head	I'd like to eat whatever I want, whenever I want it

KEEP GOING TO NEXT PAGE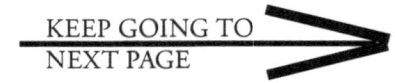

Eyebrow	But that isn't the reality of my body and my metabolism
Side of Eye	I am open to learning to tap before eating any snack foods
Under the Eye	I am open to changing my habits
Nose	I'd rather deal with whatever emotion I'm trying to feed
Chin	Instead of hurting my body
Collarbone	I can change this pattern one bite at a time
Under the Arm	I have the tools
Top of Head	I just need to use them

 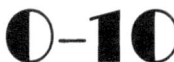 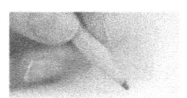

"Mindfulness isn't difficult, we just need to remember to do it." - Sharon Salzberg

92

I don't have time to exercise.

The Setup

I don't have time to exercise. I'm a very busy person. Where would I find the time? I have way too many things to do so I don't think I really have the time to exercise. In spite of all of my excuses about exercise, I choose to love and accept myself anyway. Even though I have an amazing number of excuses about why I don't have time to exercise, I honor the part of me that knows I really do.

The Tapping

Eyebrow	I don't have time to exercise
Side of Eye	Sometimes that feels really true
Under the Eye	Sometimes I know it is just an excuse
Nose	I am really busy
Chin	I have a lot on my plate
Collarbone	Other people rely upon me to get things done
Under the Arm	I often feel overwhelmed with all I have to do
Top of Head	Let's face it, adding exercise to the mix seems pretty overwhelming

KEEP GOING TO NEXT PAGE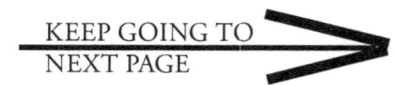

Eyebrow	At the very least it could be quite inconvenient
Side of Eye	I don't know how I would fit it into my day
Under the Eye	What other things would I have to give up?
Nose	If I get other people to do their own stuff I probably could find some time to exercise but that will mean conflict
Chin	If I asked for help with some of my own stuff I probably could find some time to exercise
Collarbone	I don't have to do it all at once
Under the Arm	I could do a little bit at a time, like just parking one spot farther out in the parking lot
Top of Head	If I really wanted to exercise I could be creative in my scheduling

   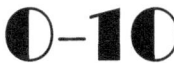   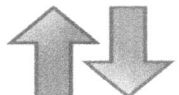

Eyebrow	The first step is deciding I really want to do this
Side of Eye	Then I can decide what exercise or exercises I want to do
Under the Eye	It might be fun to take a class and learn something new
Nose	I could get the whole family involved some of the time
Chin	Or I could save some of this time as "me time"
Collarbone	It feels good to think about doing this for myself
Under the Arm	I have the same amount of time each day that everyone else does
Top of Head	It is up to me to decide how to use it

   0-10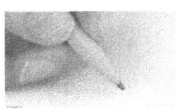

Today I faced the marshmallow fluff, and I lost.

The Setup

Even though I gave into temptation and ate marshmallow fluff by the spoonful today, I deeply and completely love and accept myself anyway. Even though I ate marshmallow fluff in response to being tired and frustrated, I choose to view myself with love and compassion. Even though I ate marshmallow fluff in secret so nobody would know, I choose to get back on track right now.

The Tapping

Eyebrow	I ate marshmallow fluff
Side of Eye	First I put some on my brownie
Under the Eye	Then I ate some on a spoon with peanut butter
Nose	Then I just ate if off of a spoon by itself
Chin	Knowing that I still have these behaviors makes me feel so defeated sometimes
Collarbone	I wasn't really hungry but I was craving something sweet
Under the Arm	It was here, easy, and easy to hide
Top of Head	I didn't eat enough to do a lot of damage to my diet

KEEP GOING TO NEXT PAGE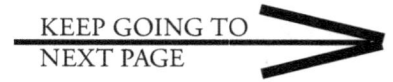

Eyebrow	But I did damage my confidence
Side of Eye	I also know that once I start, it is sometimes hard to stop
Under the Eye	It's good to know I can tap on that issue too if I need to
Nose	I'm angry with myself for eating the fluff
Chin	I'm disappointed with myself for eating the fluff
Collarbone	I feel like a failure
Under the Arm	I feel like a fraud
Top of Head	The fluff won, and I hate that

 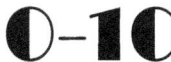 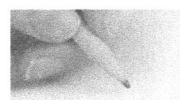

Tapping Exercise:

While tapping through the points, describe your most embarrassing food moment.

But I am still hungry.

The Setup

I am still hungry. I want to eat more food. It was really good. Of course I want more of it, and I am still hungry. A part of me knows that I am not really hungry. Another part of me wants to eat and eat and eat. Even though that part of me wants to continue eating, I choose to listen to the part that knows I don't really need that much food. Even though I feel like I am still hungry, I choose to stop eating long enough to decide what I really should do next.

The Tapping

Eyebrow	I'm still hungry
Side of Eye	I want a second portion of everything
Under the Eye	And then I want dessert
Nose	I want to keep eating
Chin	It was really good
Collarbone	I want to keep eating
Under the Arm	Just one little portion really wasn't enough to satisfy me
Top of Head	I feel like I am really hungry

KEEP GOING TO NEXT PAGE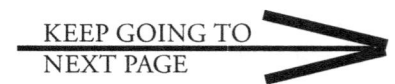

Eyebrow	Other people are getting seconds
Side of Eye	Some people are eating thirds
Under the Eye	Why not me?
Nose	Am I really hungry?
Chin	Is my eating just becoming a habit?
Collarbone	How much would it take for me to stop feeling hungry right now?
Under the Arm	I have probably already eaten enough to satisfy my body
Top of Head	I am open to clarity and guidance to help me eat only what my body really needs and can use

 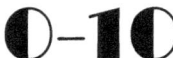 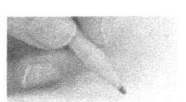

"Each patient carries his own doctor inside him." - Norman Cousins

95

A salad isn't really a meal.

The Setup

Even though I believe that a salad isn't really a meal, I deeply and completely love and accept myself - even that belief. Even though it feels like salad isn't really a whole meal, I love and accept myself anyway. Even though it feels like salad isn't really a meal, I am open to learning a new way of thinking.

The Tapping

Eyebrow	A salad doesn't feel like a meal
Side of Eye	I'm not sure why I feel that way
Under the Eye	Salad seems like a side dish
Nose	When I think of salad, I think of lettuce
Chin	I know there are other kinds of salads
Collarbone	But that isn't what pops into my head when I hear the word
Under the Arm	A salad just does not feel like a meal
Top of Head	But I choose to remain open to feeling differently in the future

 **0-10**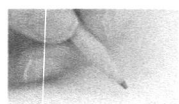

96

A donut would be really good right now.

The Setup

Even though a donut sounds really good right now, I choose to stick to my healthy eating plan. Even though a donut would really taste good to me, it has other health effects that I don't really want. Even though I want a donut right now, I love and accept myself and all of my cravings.

The Tapping

Eyebrow	A donut would be good right now
Side of Eye	I would really like a donut right now
Under the Eye	I am craving something soft and sweet
Nose	If I am perfectly honest
Chin	I am craving the comfort that I associate with donuts
Collarbone	Just as much as I am craving the taste
Under the Arm	I am open to clarity about this craving
Top of Head	I release this craving

0-10

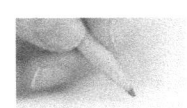

I can't go to a movie without eating a snack.

The Setup

Everyone gets snacks at the movie theater. They have popcorn, hot dogs, candy, nachos, pop, and many other things. I can't imagine going to the movie without having something to snack on. Even though I know that these snacks are not good for me, I am doing the best I can and am open to guidance. Even though I have eaten these snacks when I have gone to the movies before, I choose to forgive myself for my irresponsible behavior. Even though I don't think I could possibly enjoy the experience of going to the movie theater without eating, I love and accept myself anyway.

The Tapping

Eyebrow	I can't go to a movie without eating
Side of Eye	I really can't go to a movie without eating snacks
Under the Eye	Why would I want to?
Nose	I could see it if I couldn't afford the snacks
Chin	I can't imagine doing it on purpose
Collarbone	That would take all of the fun out of it
Under the Arm	Overpaying for high priced snacks is fun
Top of Head	It's part of the whole experience

KEEP GOING TO NEXT PAGE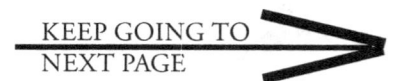

Eyebrow	At least that is what they want us to think
Side of Eye	I don't fall into that trap so much at home
Under the Eye	I don't fall into that trap at work
Nose	I wonder why I choose to believe it at the theater
Chin	That doesn't make much sense
Collarbone	My goal is really the same at either place. I want to be healthy and feel good
Under the Arm	I don't need to eat automatically. I can make the choice
Top of Head	I am open to guidance about this dilemma

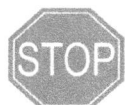 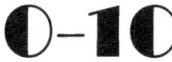 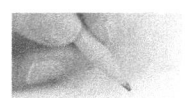

"I don't understand why asking people to eat a well-balanced, vegetarian diet is considered drastic, while it is medically conservative to cut people open." - Dean Ornish

I am deeply ashamed of how out of control I am about food.

The Setup

I am so ashamed of my inability to control my eating. Even when I am eating, my brain and inner self are often telling me to stop. But I am out of control. Something takes over and I just keep eating and eating and eating. In spite of being like an out of control animal about food, I want to let go of the shame and guilt about this situation. Even though I have shame and guilt about my eating habits at times, I am trying to learn new skills and new ways of relating to food. I get out of control around food and I am ashamed of my lack of control. Even with this character flaw of mine, I choose to take baby steps to regain a healthier way of eating and living with food.

The Tapping

Eyebrow	I am ashamed of my eating
Side of Eye	I am out of control
Under the Eye	I should be able to control my eating better
Nose	I should be able to control myself better
Chin	It's not like I don't know any better
Collarbone	I blame myself for this
Under the Arm	I'm supposed to be a smart person
Top of Head	Obviously not

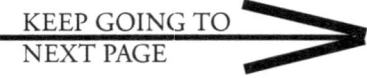

KEEP GOING TO
NEXT PAGE

Eyebrow	Other people would be appalled if they really knew how I am with food
Side of Eye	I am so ashamed of myself
Under the Eye	I'm not really out of control all the time
Nose	Just some of the time
Chin	But I am ashamed all of the time
Collarbone	That doesn't make sense
Under the Arm	I don't want to be out of control
Top of Head	I don't want to feel so much guilt and shame either

 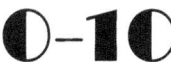 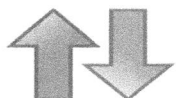

Eyebrow	I wonder if there might be something that I could change?
Side of Eye	I wonder if there is a way
Under the Eye	I could be more mindful about my eating
Nose	Feeling out of control is scary
Chin	Guilt and shame are awful
Collarbone	I would like to feel a little bit better about myself
Under the Arm	I could probably let go of these feelings at least sometimes. I can control myself when I eat a salad. I can control myself when I eat apples. That seems like a good reason to reject guilt and shame
Top of Head	I may have a bad habit of guilt and shame. I choose to stop beating myself up when it isn't appropriate

 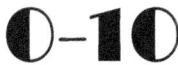 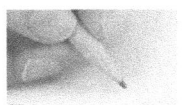

I don't want to work out tomorrow.

The Setup

Even though I don't want to work out tomorrow, I deeply and completely love and accept myself. Even though I don't want to work out tomorrow, I honor all the reasons that I might feel that way. Even though I don't want to work out tomorrow, I am hopeful that I just might change my mind.

The Tapping

Eyebrow	I don't want to work out tomorrow
Side of Eye	And tomorrow isn't even here yet
Under the Eye	How do I know how I will feel tomorrow?
Nose	What makes me think I shouldn't work out two days in a row?
Chin	That's sort of crazy
Collarbone	But the feeling is pretty strong
Under the Arm	I don't want to work out tomorrow
Top of Head	And nobody can make me

KEEP GOING TO NEXT PAGE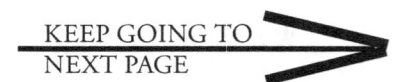

Eyebrow	That is the scary part
Side of Eye	I'm not sure I can make me either
Under the Eye	I know I will feel better if I do work out
Nose	I can choose to focus on that
Chin	I can remember how good it felt this morning
Collarbone	Or I can whine and cry about how unfair it is
Under the Arm	At this moment I'm resisting working out tomorrow
Top of Head	But I choose to let that resistance go

 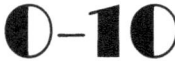 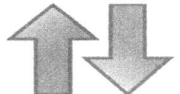

Eyebrow	I can decide tomorrow
Side of Eye	All I have to do is start
Under the Eye	That is the agreement I have with myself
Nose	Then, if I still don't want to work out
Chin	I don't have to
Collarbone	I may not want to work out right now
Under the Arm	But I'm much more hopeful about tomorrow
Top of Head	I choose to face tomorrow when it gets here

 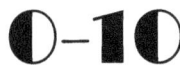 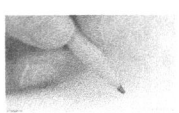

I have to use butter.

The Setup

Even though I believe I have to use butter when I cook, I love and accept myself anyway. Even though I have lots of irrational beliefs, like believing I have to use butter when I cook, I accept myself and my sometimes irrational thinking. Even though I believe I can't live without butter, I deeply and completely love and accept myself.

The Tapping

Eyebrow	I can't give up butter
Side of Eye	Everyone knows that margarine is bad for you
Under the Eye	What will I use to cook with?
Nose	What would I put on top of my toast?
Chin	How would I make frosting?
Collarbone	I just can't give up butter
Under the Arm	It doesn't matter that butter might be making me sick
Top of Head	I have to have it!

KEEP GOING TO NEXT PAGE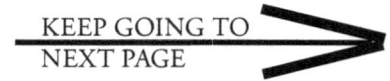

Eyebrow	No I don't
Side of Eye	Yes I do
Under the Eye	No I don't
Nose	I really don't
Chin	But I accept that I have strong attachment to eating it
Collarbone	It might be hard to find new ways to cook some of my favorite things
Under the Arm	But I know I could do it if I really try
Top of Head	I have tackled things much bigger than this successfully

 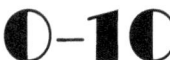 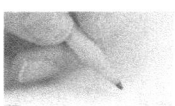

Tapping Exercise:

While tapping through the points, imagine that there has been a new law passed. Certain foods will now be prohibited. At least one of the foods on the soon-to-be-banned list is one of your favorite foods. Keep tapping while dealing with your thoughts and feelings about this upcoming event.

101

I am sick of eating salad.

The Setup

I am so sick of eating salad. If I have to eat one more salad this week I think I might vomit. Green and leafy - yuck. Why do green leafy things have to be good for me? Why can't chocolate and ice cream be just as good for me? Does anybody really like eating salads all the time? I am sick of eating salad. In spite of these very strong feelings, I deeply and completely love and accept myself anyway. Lettuce, cabbage, and spinach - Oh my. I'm just sick of it. I choose to love and accept myself anyway, including these feelings.

The Tapping

Eyebrow	Sick of salad
Side of Eye	Sick of salad
Under the Eye	Sick of salad
Nose	Did I mention that I am sick of salad?
Chin	I hate the way it looks
Collarbone	I hate the way it smells
Under the Arm	I hate the way it crunches
Top of Head	I hate the way it sounds when I chew it

KEEP GOING TO NEXT PAGE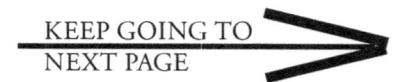

Eyebrow	I hate everything about salad right now
Side of Eye	I am sick of eating salad
Under the Eye	Nobody told me I had to eat it
Nose	I have chosen to eat it myself
Chin	I must be choosing it for a reason
Collarbone	Is that reason still valid?
Under the Arm	Could I reach my goals while eating other things too?
Top of Head	Sure I could. I can eat salad or not eat salad. It is my choice

 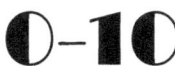 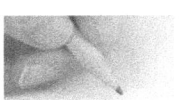

"Eating crappy food isn't a reward - - it's a punishment." - Drew Carey

Food makes me crazy.

The Setup

Even though food makes me crazy, I love and accept myself and all of my feelings about this. Even though food makes me crazy, I love and accept myself anyway. Even though food makes me crazy, I love and forgive myself for all of the craziness.

The Tapping

Eyebrow	Food makes me crazy
Side of Eye	Food makes me crazy
Under the Eye	Food makes me crazy
Nose	Food makes me crazy
Chin	Food makes me crazy
Collarbone	Food makes me crazy
Under the Arm	Food makes me crazy
Top of Head	Food makes me crazy

　　**0-10**　　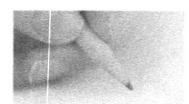

103

Diet is a 4-letter word.

The Setup

Even though I consider diet to be a 4-letter word, I love and accept myself anyway. Just hearing "diet" gives me an unpleasant feeling. I react to it pretty strongly. I just don't want to do it. Even though I am reacting strongly to that word, I choose to make my choices more rationally. Even though I consider diet to be a 4-letter word, I am open to clarity about my feelings. Even though I consider diet to be a 4-letter word, I choose to remember that love is a 4-letter word too and is perfectly acceptable to me.

The Tapping

Eyebrow	Diet is a 4-letter word
Side of Eye	And 4-letter words are all bad words aren't they?
Under the Eye	Of course not
Nose	I know lots of really good 4-letter words
Chin	Saying that diet is a bad word is another one of my excuses
Collarbone	There are better words to use to describe my eating plan
Under the Arm	I'm being pretty silly to sabotage my success based on a word
Top of Head	Diet is a 4-letter word but I choose to let go of this aversion

 **0-10**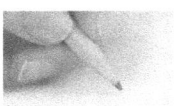

I eat when I am under stress.

The Setup

I eat when I am under stress, and boy am I under stress now. I'm not sure I can deal with all of this pressure without eating. I've got to be productive, so I've got to eat. I've got to be successful, so I've got to eat. My life is a real pressure cooker right now. Even though I have this belief that I have to eat in order to reduce my stress, I am trying to remain open to seeing other options. Even though I have had this belief that I have to eat in order to manage my stressful life, I am open to reducing my stress in other ways too. Even though I have always had this habit of eating in order to manage my stress, I deeply and completely love and accept myself, my feelings, and my beliefs.

The Tapping

Eyebrow	I am really stressed out right now
Side of Eye	And I don't think I can manage it
Under the Eye	I've always used food to manage my stress in the past
Nose	And it seems reasonable to do it again
Chin	I can't afford to let my stress
Collarbone	Interfere with my success
Under the Arm	I've got to manage it somehow
Top of Head	The stress is really mounting

KEEP GOING TO NEXT PAGE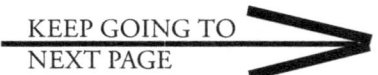

Eyebrow	And I know that I should probably find some ways to prevent some of it
Side of Eye	So that I don't feel like I have to eat so much
Under the Eye	I have all of this stress
Nose	And is seems like food makes me feel better
Chin	At least for a little while
Collarbone	This stress
Under the Arm	All of this stress
Top of Head	Feeling all of this stress

 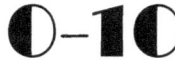 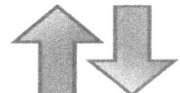

Eyebrow	I feel this stress in my body
Side of Eye	I feel this stress in my spirit
Under the Eye	I notice this stress in my words
Nose	I can see this stress in my behavior
Chin	It seems that stress management is in order
Collarbone	Eating isn't the answer
Under the Arm	I choose to look for reasonable options
Top of Head	I choose to look for multiple modes of relief

 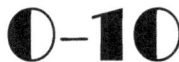 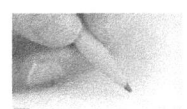

I want people to like me for who I am, not what I look like.

The Setup

I want people to like me for who I am. If I am thin, people that act like they like me may just like the way I look, not the real me. Even though I'm afraid that people won't like the real me if I lose weight, I deeply and completely love and accept myself. Even though I feel certain that people who like me now are liking the real me, I deeply and completely love and accept myself. Even though I'm afraid to lose weight, because I won't know who really likes me or not, I love and accept myself anyway.

The Tapping

Eyebrow	I guess I use my weight to screen people in or out of my life
Side of Eye	As an overweight person
Under the Eye	If they like me, I know it is for who I really am
Nose	At least I think I know that
Chin	If I were thin, they might just like me for my body
Collarbone	That would be awful
Under the Arm	I could get hurt that way
Top of Head	So I am using my weight

KEEP GOING TO NEXT PAGE
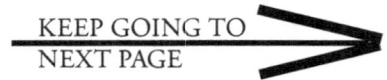

Eyebrow	To try to keep from being hurt by other people
Side of Eye	My logical brain knows that doesn't really make sense
Under the Eye	But it feels safer to me that way
Nose	I am open to understanding my feelings about this
Chin	I obviously have a friendship fear
Collarbone	I choose to overcome that fear
Under the Arm	I am afraid of getting hurt
Top of Head	I choose to overcome that fear

 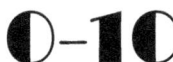 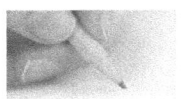

"Weight (too much or too little) is a by-product. Weight is what happens when you use food to flatten your life. Even with aching joints, it's not about food. Even with arthritis, diabetes, high blood pressure. It's about your desire to flatten your life. It's about the fact you've given up without saying so." - Geneen Roth

I want more food.

The Setup

Even though I really want more food right now, I love and accept myself. Even though I really want more food right now, I deeply and completely love and accept myself. Even though I really want more food right now, I love and accept myself anyway.

The Tapping

Eyebrow	I want more food
Side of Eye	I want more food
Under the Eye	I want more food
Nose	I want more food
Chin	I want more food
Collarbone	I want more food
Under the Arm	I want more food
Top of Head	I want more food

KEEP GOING TO NEXT PAGE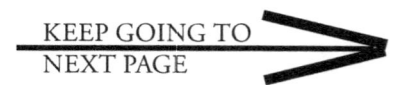

Eyebrow	If a little is good, a lot has got to be better
Side of Eye	I want more food
Under the Eye	If a little makes me feel better, a lot would make me feel great
Nose	I want more food
Chin	I want more food
Collarbone	No small portions for me
Under the Arm	I want more food
Top of Head	No medium portions for me

 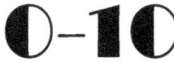 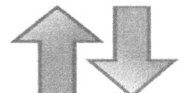

Eyebrow	I want more food
Side of Eye	I can't seem to be satisfied with a small amount
Under the Eye	I can't seem to be satisfied at all
Nose	I want more food
Chin	I want more food
Collarbone	Give me more food
Under the Arm	I want more food
Top of Head	I want more food

 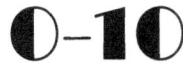 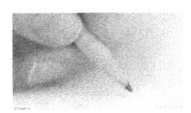

It's time to exercise, and I don't want to.

The Setup

Even though it is time to exercise right now, and I don't want to, I honor and respect my thoughts about this. Even though it is time to exercise right now, and I don't want to, I honor and respect my feelings about this. Even though it is time to exercise right now, and I don't want to, I honor and respect myself anyway.

The Tapping

Eyebrow	It is time to exercise
Side of Eye	And I don't want to
Under the Eye	That's okay
Nose	I don't always have to want to do something
Chin	There might be a good reason
Collarbone	And I am open to clarity
Under the Arm	This might also be an excuse
Top of Head	And I am open to clarity

KEEP GOING TO NEXT PAGE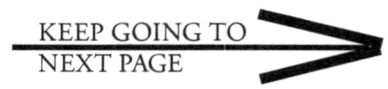

Eyebrow	This might be self-sabotage
Side of Eye	And I am open to clarity
Under the Eye	Not wanting to do something isn't such a big deal
Nose	I can choose to exercise right now anyway
Chin	Or I can choose to exercise a little later
Collarbone	I can listen to my inner guidance and decide if I will exercise or not
Under the Arm	I choose to make this decision with love and respect for my feelings
Top of Head	I choose to make this decision with love and respect for myself

 **0–10**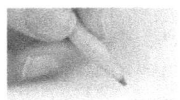

Tapping Exercise:

Set a timer for 5 minutes. Spend the entire 5 minutes tapping through the points. Let your mind wander. If a topic catches your attention, focus on it for as long as feels necessary then allow your mind to wander again.

I must clean my plate.

The Setup

I have a compulsion to eat whatever is on my plate. Leaving food seems like a waste. I'd like to say that this is why I am a member of the clean plate club, but I'm not sure that it tells the whole story. Leaving food on my plate makes me feel anxious and there really is a compulsion to finish it. I've continued to eat food, even when I don't really like it and my stomach already hurts from eating too much. Even though I have a compulsion to eat, I am open to clarity in my thinking about this. Even though I have a compulsion to eat until it is gone, I am open to embracing my feelings about this. Even though I have a habit of eating everything on my plate, no matter what, I choose to love and accept myself deeply, completely, and without reservation.

The Tapping

Eyebrow	My food compulsion
Side of Eye	My finish the whole plate compulsion
Under the Eye	This eat the whole bowl habit
Nose	This need to eat it all
Chin	This intense need to finish the whole thing
Collarbone	This food compulsion
Under the Arm	This leftover food anxiety
Top of Head	I must eat it all

KEEP GOING TO NEXT PAGE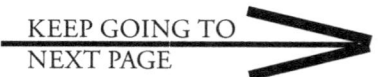

Eyebrow	Anxiety about leaving food on my plate
Side of Eye	This compulsion to eat food
Under the Eye	I must eat it all
Nose	The feeling is so strong
Chin	But I am open to clarity
Collarbone	The feeling is so intense
Under the Arm	And I choose to remain open to new ways of feeling
Top of Head	I choose to accept my thoughts, feelings, and behaviors

 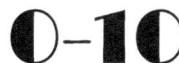 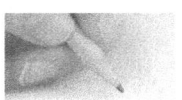

"By choosing healthy over skinny you are choosing self-love over self-judgment. You are beautiful!" - Steve Maraboli

Stuffing the anger.

The Setup

Anger can be a scary emotion for me. I learned a long time ago that it was safer to stuff anger than to express it. I'm not sure that the lesson I learned was very accurate though. Now I don't just stuff the anger, I also stuff the food when I feel angry. Then, I still feel angry. I've just added anger toward myself to the anger list. That can't be a very good thing for anybody. I'd like to learn to handle anger more constructively. I'd like to be able to address my anger directly rather than stuff it deep inside by eating lots of food. Even though I have the habit of stuffing food and anger together, I choose to be amazed at how easy it can be to let go of this habit.

The Tapping

Eyebrow	Anger scares me
Side of Eye	Other people's anger scares me
Under the Eye	My anger scares me
Nose	I literally try to stuff it whenever I'm faced with anger
Chin	Somewhere along the way it became too difficult to stuff
Collarbone	So I added food along with the emotions
Under the Arm	That usually seems to work for a little while
Top of Head	Until I get angry with myself for overeating

KEEP GOING TO NEXT PAGE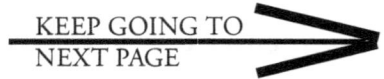

Eyebrow	Or eating the wrong things
Side of Eye	Even though anger has been a difficult emotion for me
Under the Eye	I choose to remember that things have changed in my life
Nose	Even though anger wasn't always a safe emotion for me
Chin	I choose to remember that I'm not a vulnerable child anymore
Collarbone	Even though I have this anger hang-up
Under the Arm	I am open to learning new ways to receive it and express it
Top of Head	I choose to let go of this habit of stuffing anger and food

 **0-10**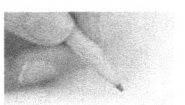

Tapping Exercise:

Begin tapping. Remember a time when expressing your feelings was a problem. What feeling were you expressing? To whom were you expressing it? What was their reaction? When you think about that event now, what thoughts or feelings come up? When do those same feelings show up in your life now?

The Christmas cookies are calling me.

The Setup

Those Christmas cookies are calling my name. "Eat me!" I'm sure you must hear them. I'm feeling powerless to resist and that bothers me somewhat. On the other hand, there is a part of me that hopes I will give in. That conflict between giving in and resisting takes an awful lot of energy. Even though I feel like the cookies are calling me, I choose to remember that I have options. Even though a part of me wants to give in, I choose to remember my long term plans. Even though a part of me wants to resist, I choose to remember that one cookie wouldn't be such a bad thing. I have choices. I have power. I love and accept myself, no matter which choice I make.

The Tapping

Eyebrow	Those Christmas cookies
Side of Eye	I really want one, or two, or twelve
Under the Eye	That is the problem
Nose	I'm not sure I can stop at just one
Chin	And if I give in to one
Collarbone	I'm likely to eat the whole batch
Under the Arm	One cookie would make me feel good
Top of Head	Several would make me feel sick

KEEP GOING TO
NEXT PAGE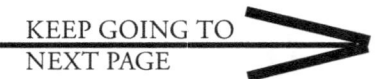

Eyebrow	And a whole batch would make me feel like a failure
Side of Eye	Cookies don't really talk
Under the Eye	They aren't calling me
Nose	I am choosing to focus on the fact that they exist
Chin	That is a choice I am making
Collarbone	I could get busy with something else
Under the Arm	They will still be there later
Top of Head	It's not a choice I have to make right now

 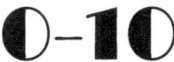 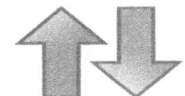

Eyebrow	It might be interesting to see if I still hear them after a warm bath
Side of Eye	Do I still hear them after a good workout?
Under the Eye	Are they as loud if I am playing a game?
Nose	Cookies can't control me
Chin	Sounds like I'm worried that I can't control me either
Collarbone	Either decision I make is okay
Under the Arm	I choose to love myself, with or without the cookies
Top of Head	I choose to accept myself, with or without cookies

 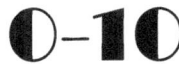 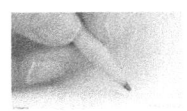

I never feel satisfied.

The Setup

Even though I never seem to feel satisfied after I eat, I deeply and completely love and accept myself. Even though I never seem to feel satisfied after a meal, I deeply and completely love and accept myself anyway. Even though I never seem to feel satisfied after eating a meal, I deeply and completely love and accept myself and all of my feelings.

The Tapping

Eyebrow	I don't feel satisfied
Side of Eye	I don't feel satisfied
Under the Eye	I don't feel satisfied
Nose	I don't feel satisfied
Chin	I don't feel satisfied
Collarbone	I don't feel satisfied
Under the Arm	I don't feel satisfied
Top of Head	I don't feel satisfied

KEEP GOING TO NEXT PAGE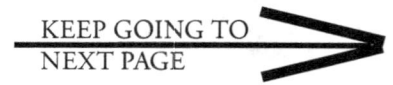

Eyebrow	Since I just finished a meal, it can't have anything to do with hunger
Side of Eye	Since I just finished a meal, it can't really have anything to do with food
Under the Eye	I am open to learning what this is really about
Nose	Even though I don't feel satisfied right now
Chin	I am open to discovering what could make me feel differently
Collarbone	Even though I don't feel completely satisfied right now
Under the Arm	I choose to look for ways to feel better
Top of Head	I choose to wait patiently until satisfaction is a reality for me

 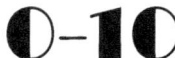 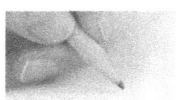

"Usually, we believe that our pain is a misfortune that needs to be fixed, but in fact, all pain (physical, mental, and emotional) is a necessary step towards becoming conscious. " Eliza Mada Dalian

112

I am sick of my body.

The Setup

Even though I am sick of my body, I choose to love and accept myself anyway. Even though I am sick of my body and can't even stand to look at it, I choose to love and accept myself anyway. Even though I am sick of my body, I choose to love and accept myself anyway.

The Tapping

Eyebrow	I am sick of my body
Side of Eye	I am sick of my body
Under the Eye	I am sick of my body
Nose	I am sick of my body
Chin	I am sick of my body
Collarbone	I am sick of my body
Under the Arm	I am sick of my body
Top of Head	I am sick of my body

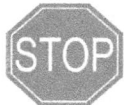   **0-10**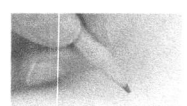

113

I am too impatient to really be successful.

The Setup

Patience is a virtue, or so they say. What do they know about it? When it comes to dieting, I'm definitely impatient. I want results right now. If I eat well at one meal, I want it to show up on the scales within an hour, or at least by the next day. My head knows that is unrealistic, but it is really what I want. That is my feeling about it. When I can't see results right away it is easy for me to give up. I think I am too impatient to really be successful with weight loss.

The Tapping

Eyebrow	This impatience about weight loss
Side of Eye	This impatience about weight loss
Under the Eye	This impatience about weight loss
Nose	This impatience about weight loss
Chin	This impatience about weight loss
Collarbone	This impatience about weight loss
Under the Arm	This impatience about weight loss
Top of Head	This impatience about weight loss

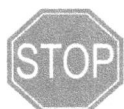 **0–10**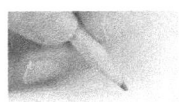

I am afraid I will stay fat forever.

The Setup

I am afraid that I will stay fat forever. I don't believe I could take that. I hate being fat. Staying fat means that I will always hate myself too. I accept my thoughts about this. I accept my feelings about this. I choose to believe that my thoughts and feelings could change.

The Tapping

Eyebrow	I am afraid that I will stay fat forever
Side of Eye	And I just don't think I can stand that
Under the Eye	Being fat is bad
Nose	I'm fat
Chin	That makes me bad too
Collarbone	Being fat is disgusting
Under the Arm	I'm fat
Top of Head	That makes me disgusting too

KEEP GOING TO NEXT PAGE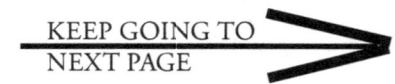

Eyebrow	Being fat is shameful
Side of Eye	I'm fat
Under the Eye	That makes me shameful too
Nose	I'm afraid that it will be like this forever
Chin	This isn't the future I want
Collarbone	I am so glad that I can tap about these thoughts
Under the Arm	I am so glad that I can tap about these feelings
Top of Head	I claim my own worth and power - right now. I can take action and stop worrying about the future

 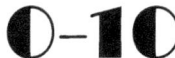 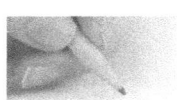

"No matter what we weigh, those of us who are compulsive eaters have anorexia of the soul." - Geneen Roth

I want the entire bag of chips, not one or two.

The Setup

Even though I want the entire bag of chips, I love and accept myself. Even though I want the entire bag of chips, I love and accept myself. Even though I want the entire bag of chips, I deeply and completely love and accept myself.

The Tapping

Eyebrow	I want the entire bag of chips
Side of Eye	I know one or two would be okay
Under the Eye	But I don't want to have to stop with just two
Nose	I want the entire bag
Chin	Or at least I want to eat until I feel like stopping
Collarbone	I don't want to control myself
Under the Arm	I want to eat uncontrollably
Top of Head	I want the entire bag of chips

KEEP GOING TO NEXT PAGE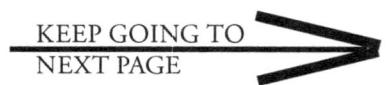

Eyebrow	I could never be satisfied with just one
Side of Eye	I want the feeling of eating a ton of chips
Under the Eye	I want to gorge myself
Nose	I want the salt
Chin	I want the grease
Collarbone	I want the calories
Under the Arm	I want to get fat
Top of Head	I want high blood pressure

 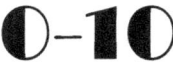 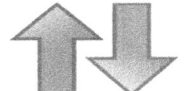

Eyebrow	And the chips are worth that
Side of Eye	Well, maybe not
Under the Eye	I am open to finding another way to get the feeling I crave
Nose	I wonder if the third chip tastes as good as the first one
Chin	I could probably stop when I notice that they are not tasting as good anymore if I eat those chips slowly
Collarbone	I could learn how many chips are the right amount for me
Under the Arm	It could be 100, 20, 2, or 0
Top of Head	I choose to listen to my body on this one and trust that it knows how many I can handle

 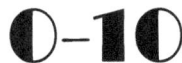 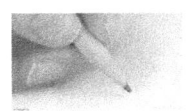

If I lose too much weight I'll have too much hanging skin to ever look good.

The Setup

I'm afraid of what my body will look like if I lose too much weight. I'll probably have skin hanging everywhere. That will look even worse than being fat. Even though I have these fears, I deeply and completely love and accept myself. My stomach will sag. My arms will get floppy, and my thighs will jiggle. Even though I'm afraid of what my body will look like if I lose weight, I deeply and completely love and accept myself anyway.

The Tapping

Eyebrow	I'm afraid of what my body will look like if I lose weight
Side of Eye	I'll probably look worse than I do right now
Under the Eye	I'm afraid of having lots of hanging skin
Nose	My stomach will sag
Chin	My arms will get floppy
Collarbone	My thighs will jiggle
Under the Arm	So I probably should just stay fat
Top of Head	I worry about what my body will look like if I continue losing weight

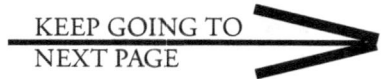

KEEP GOING TO NEXT PAGE

Eyebrow	I guess I'm a worrier
Side of Eye	I would prefer to have a firm body
Under the Eye	But I'll have to exercise for that
Nose	It's true that it could be a lot of work to tone up since I've been overweight for such a long time
Chin	But I could do it if it is really important to me
Collarbone	I could even get plastic surgery if I really wanted to
Under the Arm	I really do have a lot of choices
Top of Head	I'll have more choices if I am thin than I will if I am fat

 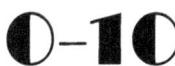 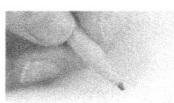

Tapping Exercise:

Look in the mirror and view your chest. Look at it from the side and from the front. What do you see? What words pop into your head. Tap about any negative thoughts or feelings that arise.

117

This candy bar is my reward.

The Setup

Even though I always get a candy bar as my reward, I deeply love and accept myself. Even though I always get a candy bar as my reward, and I definitely deserve a reward, I love and accept myself anyway. Even though I think I will feel cheated if I don't get a reward right now, I love and accept myself.

The Tapping

Eyebrow	This candy bar is my reward for grocery shopping
Side of Eye	I always get something
Under the Eye	Sometimes it is chocolate
Nose	And sometimes I get something peppermint
Chin	It can be a variety of things
Collarbone	But I always get something
Under the Arm	It is a reward for a job well done
Top of Head	I don't know where I learned that there has to be a candy reward for grocery shopping

KEEP GOING TO NEXT PAGE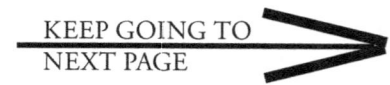

Eyebrow	I don't really even mind going to the grocery
Side of Eye	Carrying the groceries into the house can be a bit of a task
Under the Eye	I wonder if there are some other feelings about the grocery shopping that I need to address
Nose	It would be a shame to blow my diet with candy if there is something else really bothering me
Chin	Saying that I have to get a reward does sound true
Collarbone	So does saying that I resent having to do it all by myself
Under the Arm	I should probably tap on both issues
Top of Head	I can choose the candy bar or I can choose not to. It is up to me

 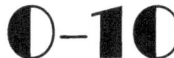 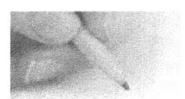

"We should resolve now that the health of this nation is a national concern; that financial barriers in the way of attaining health shall be removed; that the health of all it's citizens deserves the help of all the nation." - Harry S. Truman

I hate deciding what to cook for dinner.

The Setup

I hate deciding what to cook for dinner. Even when I plan my menu ahead, sometimes I'm just too tired to cook a healthy, nutritious meal. I accept myself, my tiredness, and my indecision as part of who I am right now. I choose to believe that even this can change.

The Tapping

Eyebrow	I hate deciding what to cook for dinner
Side of Eye	Not only that, but I'm often too tired to cook when I get home
Under the Eye	That wouldn't be a problem if I would just skip the meal
Nose	Or snack on some vegetables
Chin	But when I'm tired I seem to reach for the sweet or salty snack foods
Collarbone	I would tell everyone else to just not have those foods in the house
Under the Arm	But I will still tend to overeat other foods too
Top of Head	I would rather address the real problem

KEEP GOING TO
NEXT PAGE
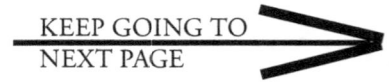

Eyebrow	I'm just not sure what the real problem is
Side of Eye	I am open to understanding what is going on with me
Under the Eye	I am open to changing my patterns
Nose	I really don't have to do this all alone
Chin	I could ask for help
Collarbone	I could ask for support
Under the Arm	I might still reach for sweet or salty snacks sometimes
Top of Head	But if I could eat more healthy even one night a week it would be worth it

 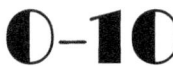 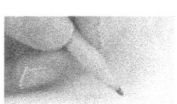

Tapping Exercise:

Begin tapping. Describe an embarrassing clothing event from your past.

I've lost the same 5 pounds at least 20 times in my life.

The Setup

It seems that I've lost the same 5 pounds at least 20 times in my life. Heck, I've lost that 5 pounds at least 4 times in the last 2 months. This is getting old fast. Even though I am frustrated with the ups and downs of my weight, I choose to remain focused and calm. Even though I am frustrated with the ups and downs of my weight, I choose not to fall into a pattern of helplessness or despair. Even though I am frustrated with the ups and downs of my weight, I deeply and completely love and accept myself anyway.

The Tapping

Eyebrow	My weight is up
Side of Eye	My weight is down
Under the Eye	Each time it zooms back up I get discouraged
Nose	Each time it creeps back down I'm also discouraged because it is so slow
Chin	I want it to be easy
Collarbone	I want it to be continuous
Under the Arm	I don't want to struggle with it
Top of Head	I don't really want to take responsibility for it

KEEP GOING TO
NEXT PAGE

Eyebrow	I know my metabolism is working against me
Side of Eye	But I'm not necessarily helping things either
Under the Eye	At least if my weight goes up
Nose	I usually get it to go back down
Chin	That is a good thing
Collarbone	I would do well to remember to be thankful for even the small improvements
Under the Arm	I've done this to my body over a lifetime
Top of Head	Managing my weight will also be a lifetime activity

 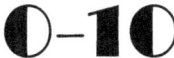 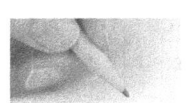

"Eat healthily, sleep well, breathe deeply, move harmoniously." - Jean-Pierre Barral

My daily schedule revolves around food.

The Setup

Even though my daily schedule seems to revolve around food, I choose to look for other ways to structure my day. Even though my thoughts continually turn to food, I choose to redirect my attention to thoughts and activities that will be healthier for me. Even though I seem to organize my schedule around mealtime, I choose to be patient with myself while I am changing.

The Tapping

Eyebrow	My daily schedule revolves around food
Side of Eye	That is more than a little bit disturbing to me
Under the Eye	I was driving to an appointment and worried about when I would get breakfast
Nose	That wouldn't be so bad, but there was plenty of time
Chin	My appointment was early
Collarbone	I wasn't even hungry
Under the Arm	I pulled through the drive-through for breakfast, just in case
Top of Head	That kind of obsessive thinking makes me feel crazy

KEEP GOING TO NEXT PAGE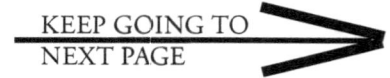

Eyebrow	I let thoughts and worries about food ruin my day
Side of Eye	I let thoughts and worries about food ruin my health
Under the Eye	I let thoughts and worries about food ruin my life
Nose	It is time to change that pattern
Chin	I've changed other patterns
Collarbone	It usually isn't easy, but it is worth it in the end
Under the Arm	Even when the thoughts pop into my head, I can choose to ignore them
Top of Head	Or I can take an alternate action

 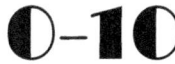 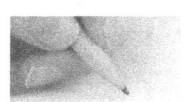

"Respect your body. Eat well. Dance forever." - Eliza Gaynor Minden

No perfect time to work out.

The Setup

Even though it feels like there is no perfect time to work out, I deeply and completely love and accept myself. Even though it is hard to get out of bed in the morning to work out, I choose to remember how good I feel when I've followed through with that plan. Even though I think I'm too tired to work out when I get home in the evening, I choose to remember how much better I sleep when I've exercised during the day. I deeply and completely love and accept myself, even when I make excuses to avoid exercise.

The Tapping

Eyebrow	There is no perfect time to work out
Side of Eye	It seems like it is too hard in the morning
Under the Eye	Because I am too sleepy
Nose	It seems like it is too hard in the evening
Chin	Because I am tired from work
Collarbone	I seem to have an excuse no matter what
Under the Arm	When I feel too sleepy in the morning
Top of Head	I choose to remember how proud of myself I feel when I follow through with the plan

KEEP GOING TO
NEXT PAGE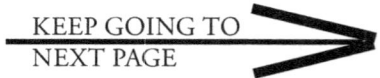

Eyebrow	When I feel too tired after work
Side of Eye	I could choose to remember how much better I sleep if I've been physically active
Under the Eye	There really is no perfect time to work out
Nose	Because any time is the perfect time to work out
Chin	What is important is that I do it
Collarbone	Not when I do it
Under the Arm	I choose to remember how good exercise makes my body feel
Top of Head	I choose to remember how good exercise is for my brain

 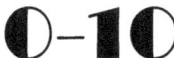 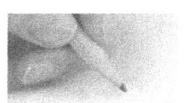

"Suffering usually relates to wanting things to be different from the way they are." - Allan Lokos

I am hungry and all I can think about is food.

The Setup

Even though I am hungry and all I can think about is food, I deeply and completely love and accept myself anyway. Even though I am hungry and all I can think about is food, I deeply and completely love and accept myself. Even though I am hungry and all I can think about is food, I am open to loving and accepting myself completely.

The Tapping

Eyebrow	I am hungry
Side of Eye	All I can think about is food
Under the Eye	I am hungry
Nose	All I can think about is food
Chin	I am hungry
Collarbone	All I can think about is food
Under the Arm	I am hungry
Top of Head	All I can think about is food

 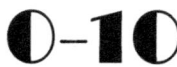 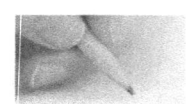

123

I don't like to waste food.

The Setup

I don't like to waste food, so I ate way too much. Even though I ate too much because I don't like to waste food, I love and accept myself completely. Even though wasting food seems very wrong, I am trying to love and accept myself. Even though I sometimes eat too much and feel like I need to eat too much so that I don't waste food, I love and accept myself anyway.

The Tapping

Eyebrow	I eat too much
Side of Eye	To avoid wasting food
Under the Eye	I eat too much
Nose	So that I don't waste food
Chin	I would rather eat too much
Collarbone	Than let food go to waste
Under the Arm	I eat too much
Top of Head	So that I don't waste food

   0-10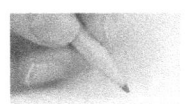

124

Once I start eating, I just can't stop.

The Setup

I feel anxious about being around food, particularly my favorite foods, because I can't trust myself to stop eating once I have started. One spoon of ice cream means I have to eat the whole thing. One cookie means I have to eat them all. Even though I have this anxiety about being around food, I want to love and accept myself anyway.

The Tapping

Eyebrow	I feel anxious about food
Side of Eye	I don't trust myself to stop once I have started
Under the Eye	That is a very uncomfortable feeling
Nose	I would like to eat more normally
Chin	Small, satisfying portions
Collarbone	Just a taste of this and a bite of that
Under the Arm	But I haven't been able to do that in the past
Top of Head	And I don't believe I can do it in the future either

KEEP GOING TO NEXT PAGE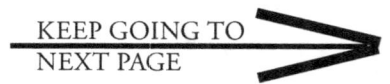

Eyebrow	Every time I try - I fail
Side of Eye	Food is everywhere
Under the Eye	It makes me feel somewhat crazy
Nose	I want to have a more normal relationship with food
Chin	I'd like to be able to trust myself too
Collarbone	Truth is - the first bite is the best
Under the Arm	Continuing to eat just doesn't bring back the same feeling as the first bite, no matter how hard I try
Top of Head	I choose to remain calm and confident when faced with food. I choose to enjoy that first bite and then stop if that fits better with my fitness goals

 **0-10**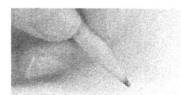

Tapping Exercise:

For the next three days, tap before each meal and snack.

Food is my only true friend.

The Setup

Food seems to be my only true friend. Everyone else has let me down at some time or not been there when I need them. At least it seems that way. In spite of this truth, I love and accept myself anyway. Even though food seems to be my only true friend, I choose to keep believing in the possibility that even this could change. I love and accept myself during this process.

The Tapping

Eyebrow	Food is my only true friend
Side of Eye	Without food, I would feel all alone
Under the Eye	Food is reliable
Nose	Food never lets me down
Chin	Food is always there when I need it
Collarbone	Food never criticizes me
Under the Arm	Food never laughs at me
Top of Head	Food never breaks its promises

KEEP GOING TO NEXT PAGE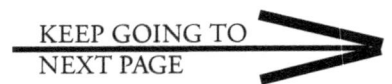

Eyebrow	Food is my only true friend
Side of Eye	Too much of a good thing can be bad though
Under the Eye	My food friend is really making me sick
Nose	My food friend sometimes makes me feel guilty or ashamed
Chin	My food friend is jealous and keeps me from making other real friends
Collarbone	My food friend may be toxic for me
Under the Arm	It might be better for me to face my friend problems rather than turning to food
Top of Head	I want to feel hopeful that I can have friends other than food in my life

 **0–10**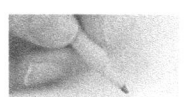

"I am not my body. My body is nothing without me." - Tom Stoppard

I can't trust my body to tell me when to stop eating.

The Setup

Even though I can't trust my body to tell me when to stop eating, I choose to try a more rational approach to eating. Even though I can't trust my body to tell me when to stop eating, I acknowledge this issue and know that I am doing the best I can. Even though I have this problem and I can't trust my body to tell me when to stop eating, I am open to the possibility that this is a temporary problem.

The Tapping

Eyebrow	I can't trust my body to tell me when to stop eating
Side of Eye	I just keep eating and eating and eating
Under the Eye	I could never trust my body to know when to stop
Nose	And if my body actually knows, it isn't telling me
Chin	Or, maybe I'm just not listening
Collarbone	How would my body tell me that it is time to stop?
Under the Arm	What signs am I looking for?
Top of Head	Maybe my body is saying I should stop, but I'm saying I should eat more

KEEP GOING TO NEXT PAGE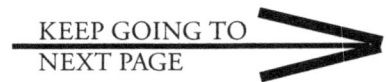

Eyebrow	That would sure be confusing
Side of Eye	Eat more
Under the Eye	Eat less
Nose	Stop eating
Chin	Don't stop eating
Collarbone	Mixed signals like that are a problem
Under the Arm	I only listen to the message I want to hear
Top of Head	Maybe I can trust my body

 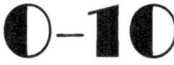 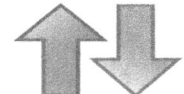

Eyebrow	I can't trust my body
Side of Eye	Yes I can
Under the Eye	I could probably pay more attention to what my body is trying to tell me
Nose	Then I would at least know I can trust my body, even if I choose not to listen
Chin	I want to learn to listen to my body's guidance and wisdom
Collarbone	My body really does know what I need
Under the Arm	I know what I need to do
Top of Head	I can trust my body. Soon my body will be able to trust me

 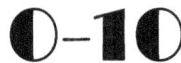 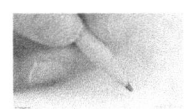

127

What if I am still unhappy even when I lose the weight?

The Setup

I have blamed my unhappiness on my weight for a very long time. What if I am still unhappy when I lose the weight? Then my unhappiness would be my own fault. Even though I am afraid I will still be unhappy when I lose the weight, I choose to move forward with hope and confidence. Even though I'm not sure how I will feel when I get to my goal weight I choose to expect pride in my accomplishment. Even though things might not be perfect when I get to my goal weight, I choose to remember that my happiness isn't tied to my weight.

The Tapping

Eyebrow	I'm afraid I will always be unhappy
Side of Eye	I've been blaming my unhappiness on my weight
Under the Eye	That has kept me from dealing with my problems
Nose	I thought that all I needed to be happy was my goal weight
Chin	I am starting to see that this might not be true
Collarbone	That scares me
Under the Arm	It hasn't really been a conscious thing until now
Top of Head	Getting to my goal weight will be a cool thing

KEEP GOING TO NEXT PAGE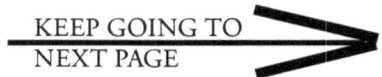

Eyebrow	But if I am realistic, I know it won't fix anything
Side of Eye	But at least I'll be facing my problems and challenges with one less issue to deal with
Under the Eye	I'm looking forward to that
Nose	I could probably start looking for solutions to my problems now
Chin	I could probably start looking for ways to be happy now
Collarbone	I don't have to lose weight in order to be happy
Under the Arm	I can choose to be happy no matter what I weigh
Top of Head	I can choose to lose weight and be happy throughout the process. I am looking forward to loving my new body

 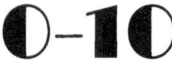 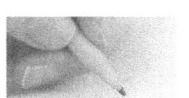

"When health is absent, wisdom cannot reveal itself, art cannot manifest, strength cannot fight, wealth becomes useless, and intelligence cannot be applied." - Herophilus

I can't exercise tonight. I have a foot injury.

The Setup

Even though I have a foot injury and obviously can't work out the way I want to, I deeply and completely love and accept myself. Even though I have a foot injury, and I'm using that as an excuse not to work out, I deeply and completely love and accept myself, even my tendency to make excuses. Even though I am using my foot injury to avoid exercising, I deeply and completely love and accept myself anyway.

The Tapping

Eyebrow	My foot hurts
Side of Eye	That makes it hard to walk on the treadmill
Under the Eye	I could ride the exercise bike
Nose	But honestly, I don't feel like doing anything
Chin	The pain in my foot all day makes me tired and grumpy
Collarbone	The last thing I feel like doing is working out
Under the Arm	I feel better when I work out
Top of Head	I feel proud of myself when I work out

KEEP GOING TO NEXT PAGE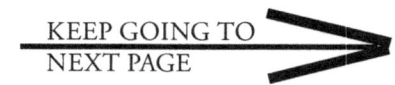

Eyebrow	My brain works better when I work out
Side of Eye	So, on some level it doesn't make sense to avoid it
Under the Eye	But I am
Nose	I can listen to my body and rest
Chin	I can keep tapping until my resistance diminishes
Collarbone	I can do both
Under the Arm	I want to find a way to honor my body and still do the things that would be healthy for me
Top of Head	I am open to guidance on what is right for me right now

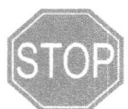 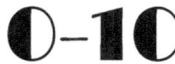 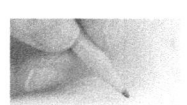

"I run because if I didn't, I'd be sluggish and glum and spend too much time on the couch. I run to breathe the fresh air. I run to explore. I run to escape the ordinary. I run... to savor the trip along the way. Life becomes a little more vibrant, a little more intense. I like that." - Dean Karnazes

I don't have to eat it all at once.

Setup

Even though I feel like I have to eat it all at once, I choose to slow down and savor the experience. Even though I feel like I have to eat it all at once, I deeply and completely love and accept myself, even my compulsion to eat. Even though I feel like I have to eat it all at once, I choose to remain calm and confident in the face of food.

The Tapping

Eyebrow	My birthday cake is really tempting me right now
Side of Eye	It isn't even done baking and I feel compelled to eat the whole thing
Under the Eye	It's almost like I think someone is going to steal it from me
Nose	So I've got to get to it first
Chin	It's my cake
Collarbone	I baked it
Under the Arm	I really don't mind sharing it with others
Top of Head	So what is the big deal?

KEEP GOING TO
NEXT PAGE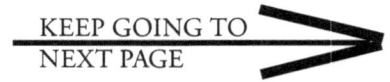

Eyebrow	When I eat too much or too fast, I don't really enjoy it
Side of Eye	This birthday cake is a masterpiece. A work of art
Under the Eye	It was made to be appreciated
Nose	Even though I am still experiencing some desire to inhale this cake
Chin	I am open to more clarity about my feelings
Collarbone	Have I confused excitement with urgency?
Under the Arm	That is a possibility
Top of Head	This won't be the last good time I'll ever have

 **0-10**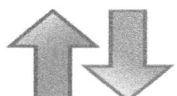

Eyebrow	When the cake is gone
Side of Eye	I can enjoy something else
Under the Eye	Sometime I will make a new one
Nose	Or I will choose something else to bake
Chin	I have lots of options
Collarbone	This cake certainly isn't the last yummy thing in my future
Under the Arm	There will be plenty of yummy things in my future
Top of Head	Probably more than I really need

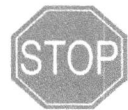 **0-10**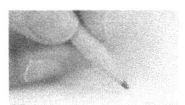

It is easier to go through the drive through than to make a salad.

The Setup

Even though I want to take the easy way out and go through that drive through for supper, I want to be able to love myself more than that. Even though it seems easier to go through the drive through than to make myself a healthy salad when I get home, I deeply and completely love and accept myself, including all of my feelings and excuses. Even though I feel like I want eating to be easy tonight, I choose to focus on loving myself, my body, and my health.

The Tapping

Eyebrow	It is easier to go through the drive through than make a salad
Side of Eye	And I want things to be easy right now
Under the Eye	I'm not sure why I don't want to make time for me tonight
Nose	Going through the drive through won't help me feel better
Chin	There are very few healthy choices there
Collarbone	And none that I can really eat right now while driving
Under the Arm	I have lots of food at home
Top of Head	Fast food is no quicker than eating an apple or a banana

KEEP GOING TO
NEXT PAGE
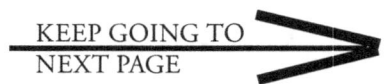

Eyebrow	So time can't be the real issue
Side of Eye	I choose to address the real issue
Under the Eye	Rather than just stuff food in my mouth
Nose	Doing that definitely won't help me
Chin	It might feel good for just a minute
Collarbone	But I am learning to enjoy food that is much more interesting than that
Under the Arm	I am worth the extra 5 minutes it might take to put together a healthy meal
Top of Head	I'm worth good, healthy, and interesting food

 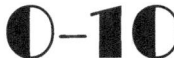 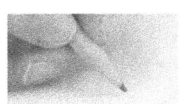

Tapping Exercise:

Watch television, read a magazine, or browse the internet. Notice the topics, images, and advertising that involve food, exercise, or body image. Which ones cause a negative emotional response for you? Tap on the thoughts and feelings that you noticed.

I look in the mirror and feel disgusted.

The Setup

Even though I feel disgusted when I see myself in the mirror, I choose to love and accept myself, even those things that I see as imperfections. Even though I feel disgust when I see myself in the mirror, I choose to be more gentle with myself and my self comments. Even though I feel disgusted when I see myself in the mirror, I choose to work toward acceptance rather than loathing.

The Tapping

Eyebrow	I don't like the way I look
Side of Eye	My sagging skin, wrinkles, and blemishes disgust me
Under the Eye	My chubbiness disgusts me
Nose	My scars disgust me
Chin	It seems that I have bought into the media view of beauty
Collarbone	And that disgusts me
Under the Arm	I know that self hatred is unhealthy
Top of Head	In fact, it keeps me from achieving health and wellness

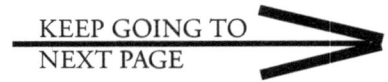

KEEP GOING TO NEXT PAGE

Eyebrow	Physical changes are inevitable
Side of Eye	I don't get a lot of say in that
Under the Eye	Other people tell me I look pretty young for my age
Nose	I could choose to believe them
Chin	I would like to see myself more accurately
Collarbone	I would also like to focus more on what I think are my better features than on those that aren't quite what I want
Under the Arm	This will take practice
Top of Head	I don't want to feel disgusted about me

 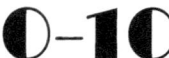 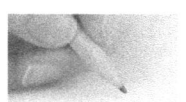

"I promise you nothing is as chaotic as it seems. Nothing is worth your health. Nothing is worth poisoning yourself into stress, anxiety, and fear." - Steve Maraboli

I want something sweet right now.

The Setup

Even though I want something sweet right now, I deeply and completely love and accept myself. Even though I want something sweet right now, and that is not part of my diet plan, I love and accept myself anyway. Even though I am strongly craving something sweet right now, I am open to clarity about this craving.

The Tapping

Eyebrow	I want something sweet right now
Side of Eye	I want something sweet right now
Under the Eye	That doesn't make a lot of sense to me
Nose	I know I am not hungry
Chin	And I don't feel particularly upset about anything
Collarbone	This craving for something sweet
Under the Arm	I am craving something sweet
Top of Head	I want something sweet

0-10

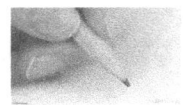

I'm having a very hard time sticking with a diet.

The Setup

Even though I'm having a very hard time sticking with a diet, I am open to feeling more confident soon. Even though I'm having a very hard time sticking with a diet, I am open to inspiration. Even though I'm having a very hard time sticking with a diet, I love and accept myself and my struggles.

The Tapping

Eyebrow	I'm having a very hard time sticking with a diet
Side of Eye	Temptation is everywhere
Under the Eye	My motivation is lacking
Nose	I'm having a very hard time
Chin	It is hard to stick with a diet
Collarbone	I'm having a hard time sticking to the diet
Under the Arm	I'm not sure I can do this
Top of Head	I'm having a very hard time sticking with a diet

   **0–10**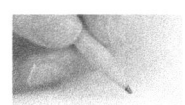

When I am stressed I want to eat.

The Setup

I'm feeling pretty stressed out. When I feel stressed I want to eat. Even though I'm feeling pretty stressed out and want to eat, I love and accept myself and all of my stress. Even though I want to eat to make myself feel better, I love and accept myself, including this impulse. Even though I want to eat right now because I'm feeling pretty stressed, I love and accept myself enough to learn other ways to relieve my stress.

The Tapping

Eyebrow	I am stressed right now
Side of Eye	And I want to eat
Under the Eye	All of this stress
Nose	I want to eat
Chin	I want my stress to go away
Collarbone	And food always helps
Under the Arm	At least for a little while
Top of Head	I am stressed right now

KEEP GOING TO NEXT PAGE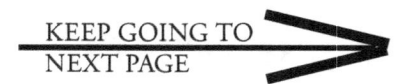

Eyebrow	So many things are bothering me
Side of Eye	And my desire to eat is building up
Under the Eye	I feel like I might lose control
Nose	I'm feeling very stressed
Chin	I am so stressed
Collarbone	That I want to eat
Under the Arm	So stressed
Top of Head	I am so stressed

   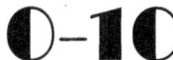   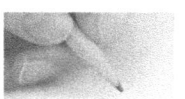

"A further sign of health is that we don't become undone by fear and trembling, but we take it as a message that it's time to stop struggling and look directly at what's threatening us." - Pema Chödrön

This plan is not working out.

The Setup

Even though I don't think this plan is really working for me, I love and accept myself anyway. Even though I don't think this plan is working out for me, I choose to remain optimistic that I can still achieve my goals. Even though I don't think this plan is working out, I love and accept myself just as I am.

The Tapping

Eyebrow	This plan is not working out
Side of Eye	And that really frustrates me
Under the Eye	This plan is not working out
Nose	And I'm afraid that I won't reach my goals
Chin	This plan is not working out
Collarbone	And that feeling is pretty uncomfortable for me
Under the Arm	This plan is not working out
Top of Head	I am frustrated and uncomfortable about that

KEEP GOING TO NEXT PAGE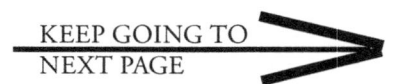

Eyebrow	This plan is not working out
Side of Eye	I am frustrated
Under the Eye	But I choose to remember that this feeling is not permanent
Nose	This plan is not working out
Chin	And I'm worried about reaching my goal
Collarbone	I acknowledge my worries and concerns
Under the Arm	This plan is not working out
Top of Head	I choose to change my plan to help me reach my goals

 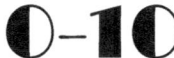 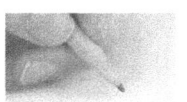

"If we are creating ourselves all the time, then it is never too late to begin creating the bodies we want instead of the ones we mistakenly assume we are stuck with." - Deepak Chopra

I blame myself for the state my body is in.

The Setup

Even though I blame myself for the state my body is in, I accept myself and my feelings. Even though I blame myself for the state my body is in, I accept myself and my thoughts. Even though I blame myself for the state my body is in, I am learning to accept all of me.

The Tapping

Eyebrow	I blame myself
Side of Eye	And I hate the state my body is in
Under the Eye	I blame myself
Nose	And I hate the state my body is in
Chin	All of this blame
Collarbone	I have all of this blame
Under the Arm	I hate my body
Top of Head	I blame myself and I hate my body

KEEP GOING TO NEXT PAGE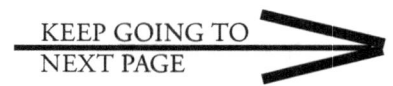

Eyebrow	It's all my fault
Side of Eye	I have nobody to blame except myself
Under the Eye	I blame myself
Nose	I hate the current state of my body
Chin	I blame myself
Collarbone	I have all of this blame
Under the Arm	My body is in bad shape
Top of Head	I have all of this blame about my body

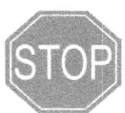 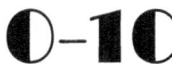 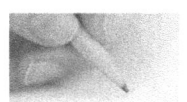

"Stop wasting so much energy hating your body; it
makes you weaker. Everything good in your life begins
from the moment you begin accepting, understanding
respecting, and loving your true self." - Harry Papas

I thought I would be at my goal weight by now.

The Setup

I thought I would be at my goal weight by now. I'm really disappointed that I didn't make it yet. I am so discouraged. Even though I thought I would be at my goal weight by now I am open to loving myself whether I ever get to that goal weight or not. Even though I thought I would already be at my goal weight by now, I choose to adjust my expectations and keep learning how to eat more healthily.

The Tapping

Eyebrow	I am not at my goal weight
Side of Eye	I wanted to be there by now
Under the Eye	I guess that was just magical thinking
Nose	It is disappointing
Chin	But its not the end of the world
Collarbone	I choose to remember that this is only a temporary setback
Under the Arm	I can still reach my goal
Top of Head	Or I can adjust my goal

KEEP GOING TO NEXT PAGE

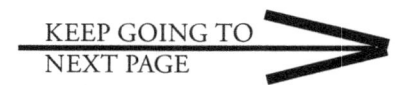

Eyebrow	I feel discouraged
Side of Eye	And I acknowledge that this feeling is real
Under the Eye	I'm also feeling guilty that I didn't do the things I needed to do
Nose	In order to be at my goal weight
Chin	Its time to re-evaluate my goal
Collarbone	And it is time to re-evaluate my methods
Under the Arm	I thought I would be at my goal weight by now but I'm not
Top of Head	I'm choosing to be okay, even with this delay in reaching my goal

 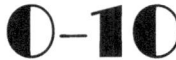 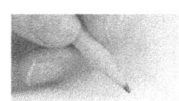

Tapping Exercise:

What are the 5 foods you can't live without? Start tapping and tell the story of your relationship with these foods.

My clothes are too tight.

The Setup

Even though my clothes are too tight and that means I'm too fat, I love and accept myself anyway. Even though my clothes are too tight, I am open to considering my options. Even though my clothes are too tight and I see that as a failure, I love and accept myself anyway.

The Tapping

Eyebrow	My clothes are too tight
Side of Eye	I don't like the way they look
Under the Eye	I don't like the way they feel
Nose	These clothes are too tight
Chin	They are very uncomfortable
Collarbone	I don't like the way my clothes look
Under the Arm	I don't like the way my clothes feel
Top of Head	Let's face it, I don't like the way I look

KEEP GOING TO NEXT PAGE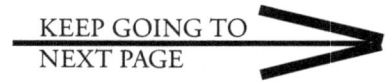

Eyebrow	And I don't like the way I feel
Side of Eye	My clothes are too tight
Under the Eye	And my body is too big
Nose	My clothes are a constant reminder of how big my body is
Chin	I want this to change
Collarbone	But I'm not sure I want to do the work to make it happen
Under the Arm	I guess I could just buy bigger clothes
Top of Head	But that seems like the easy way out

   **0-10**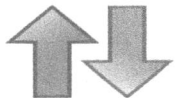

Eyebrow	Taking the easy way out doesn't feel comfortable to me
Side of Eye	My clothes are too tight
Under the Eye	My body is too big
Nose	I don't like all of these feelings
Chin	I am open to considering new options
Collarbone	My clothes are too tight
Under the Arm	I choose to accept myself anyway
Top of Head	I choose to find ways to work with what I've got to feel better now and in the future

   **0-10**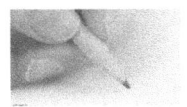

If I workout now I will be too tired to do the other things I need to do today.

The Setup

If I exercise now, I will be tired later. I can't afford to be tired later because I have a lot of things on my to do list today. Even though I'm making excuses to avoid exercise, I love and accept myself anyway. Even though I'm worried about exercise making me too tired to do the other things I need to do, I choose to treat myself with love and respect. Even though this is just another excuse in a long list of excuses I have to avoid exercise, I deeply and completely love and accept myself.

The Tapping

Eyebrow	I can't workout now
Side of Eye	I have way too much to do today
Under the Eye	If I get too tired I won't be able to get my chores done
Nose	I can't workout now
Chin	I have to conserve energy
Collarbone	I can't workout now
Under the Arm	I have too much to do
Top of Head	Working out will interfere with the rest of my day

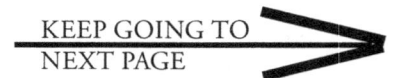

KEEP GOING TO
NEXT PAGE

Eyebrow	I can't workout now
Side of Eye	I can't workout and still get everything done
Under the Eye	I really do know that this isn't true
Nose	Moderate exercise actually gives me more energy
Chin	I am open to understanding my avoidance
Collarbone	I choose to follow my plan
Under the Arm	Even with all of my excuses
Top of Head	Of course I can work out. I can do whatever I want

   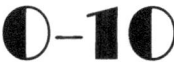   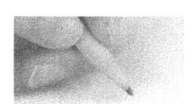

"A fit, healthy body - that is the best fashion statement." - Jess C. Scott

140

Vegetables don't taste good without cheese.

The Setup

Even though I don't think vegetables taste good without cheese, I love and accept myself anyway. Even though I don't think vegetables taste good without cheese, I deeply and completely love and accept myself. Even though I don't think vegetables taste good without cheese, I am trying to be open to new ways of thinking about this issue.

The Tapping

Eyebrow	Vegetables don't taste good without cheese
Side of Eye	Broccoli just has to have cheese
Under the Eye	Cauliflower is inedible without cheese
Nose	If I ate brussel sprouts, they would definitely require cheese
Chin	Vegetables don't taste good without cheese
Collarbone	It would be more accurate to say that some vegetables don't taste good without cheese
Under the Arm	I don't put cheese on peas
Top of Head	I don't put cheese on green beans

KEEP GOING TO NEXT PAGE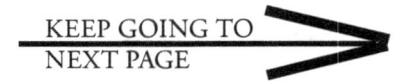

Eyebrow	I don't put cheese on carrots or celery either
Side of Eye	It might be more reasonable to say that I miss having cheese on some of my vegetables
Under the Arm	And I am stubborn enough to resist eating them in a different way
Nose	I am open to thinking about vegetables in a different way
Chin	I acknowledge my stubbornness
Collarbone	While I liked having cheese on some vegetables
Under the Arm	I am excited to think that there may be other ways
Top of Head	That are even more delicious and healthy

 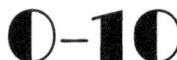 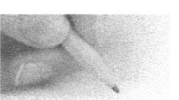

"Healthy citizens are the greatest asset any
country can have." - Winston Churchill

141

I'm worried about food.

The Setup

Even though I'm worried about food, I deeply and completely love and accept myself. As soon as I found out I was going on a trip, I started worrying about what I would eat. Seriously, that was the first thing I thought about. That seems a little bit obsessive to me. Even though I'm worried about food, I choose to calm myself down and focus on other things. I choose to allow my food choices to come easily and naturally, in spite of my food worry.

The Tapping

Eyebrow	This food worry
Side of Eye	I'm worried about food
Under the Eye	Worried about food
Nose	This food worry
Chin	I'm worried about food
Collarbone	Food worry
Under the Arm	I am worried about food
Top of Head	This food worry

   **0-10**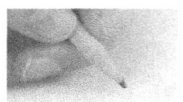

142

Abdominal workouts stink.

The Setup

Even though I believe that abdominal workouts stink, I choose to love and accept myself anyway. Even though I have always hated abdominal workouts in the past, I choose to love and accept myself anyway. I know that strengthening my core muscles is important to my overall health but I think abdominal workouts stink. In spite of this, I choose to love and accept myself anyway.

The Tapping

Eyebrow	Abdominal workouts stink
Side of Eye	Abdominal workouts stink
Under the Eye	Abdominal workouts stink
Nose	Abdominal workouts stink
Chin	Abdominal workouts stink
Collarbone	Abdominal workouts stink
Under the Arm	Abdominal workouts stink
Top of Head	Abdominal workouts stink

0-10

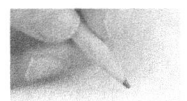

I eat food just because it is there.

The Setup

I have a tendency to eat food just because it is there, I love and accept myself, even though I have unhealthy behaviors. Even though I eat food without any real good reason, I am learning to love and accept myself anyway. Even though I eat food and I don't even know why, I choose to love and accept myself anyway.

The Tapping

Eyebrow	I seem to eat food for no good reason
Side of Eye	If it is there - I eat it
Under the Eye	I eat food even when I am not hungry
Nose	Heck, sometimes I eat food that I don't even like
Chin	My tendency to eat food just because it is available
Collarbone	Is not good for my body
Under the Arm	And when I notice what I'm doing, I feel like a failure
Top of Head	This tendency to constantly eat is not a behavior that I want to continue

KEEP GOING TO NEXT PAGE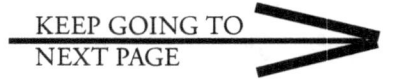

Eyebrow	I've tried to manage it by not having food around
Side of Eye	But that is not realistic for my life
Under the Eye	I can limit the choices, but it won't stop my overeating
Nose	I don't really believe that I eat food just because it is there
Chin	I believe there is another reason that I don't know yet
Collarbone	When I catch myself eating, I choose to stop and consider why
Under the Arm	There is a reason behind everything I do
Top of Head	It is up to me to figure out why; then, I can change my behavior more easily

 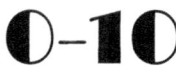 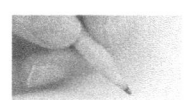

"Let food be thy medicine and medicine be thy food." - Hippocrates

I plan to follow the diet plan perfectly.

The Setup

I always plan to follow the diet perfectly. Sometimes it doesn't work out. I can usually maintain it for a few hours, days, or weeks, but then I always fail. Maybe the problem is my need to be perfect. Since I can't be perfect, I end up back where I started, or never get started at all. This pattern isn't working for me anymore. I choose to try a different way.

The Tapping

Eyebrow	I always plan to diet perfectly
Side of Eye	I always fail
Under the Eye	I am so tired of that failure
Nose	I am so discouraged
Chin	Instead of following a diet plan perfectly
Collarbone	Maybe I can try a new way
Under the Arm	Those diets are someone else's plan
Top of Head	I know a lot about diet, health, and nutrition

KEEP GOING TO NEXT PAGE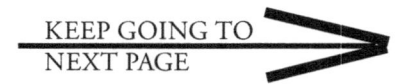

Eyebrow	I could make my own plan
Side of Eye	And follow it closely
Under the Eye	I could allow for some variation and change
Nose	Then there would be no real failure
Chin	Better yet, I could listen to my body
Collarbone	I usually listen to my emotions
Under the Arm	But my body knows what it needs and what is bad for it
Top of Head	It gives me clear signals

 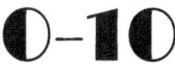 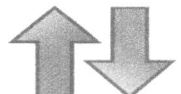

Eyebrow	I'm not perfect, so I might not always understand what my body wants and needs
Side of Eye	But I will probably get it right most of the time
Under the Eye	And that would be much better than what I'm doing to myself right now
Nose	I could view this as an experiment or an adventure
Chin	That might help me to stop thinking in terms of perfection
Collarbone	Even though I've always tried to follow the plan perfectly
Under the Arm	I haven't had a perfect plan
Top of Head	My new plan won't be perfect either and I won't follow it perfectly. I choose to love and accept myself anyway and feel proud of whatever successes I have

 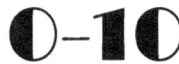 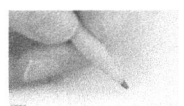

I hate having to cook a separate meal for myself.

The Setup

Even though I hate having to cook a separate meal for myself, I deeply and completely love and accept myself anyway. Even though it feels like double the work to cook my allergen free, gluten free meals and cook meals for everyone else that include all of the things I can't have, I deeply and completely love and accept myself anyway. Even though I feel resentful that other people eat what they want and I have to cook separate things for myself, I love and accept myself and choose to feel proud of myself for taking care of my body.

The Tapping

Eyebrow	I hate having to cook a separate meal for myself
Side of Eye	I guess I don't really have to
Under the Eye	I could just cook my stuff and let everyone else fend for themselves
Nose	But that just doesn't seem right
Chin	I could insist that everyone else eats the way I do
Collarbone	But that probably wouldn't work
Under the Arm	Sometimes it is hard to see a workable solution
Top of Head	In reality, most meals aren't that much of a problem

KEEP GOING TO
NEXT PAGE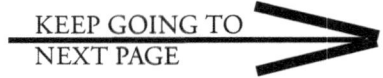

Eyebrow	But sometimes I just don't feel like dealing with it
Side of Eye	I generally end up feeling sad, mad, or resentful
Under the Eye	I don't really have to feel that way
Nose	It's just a choice I'm making
Chin	I could choose to see it another way
Collarbone	I could choose to be thankful that I've found another way of eating that is healthy for me
Under the Arm	I do get excited about finding new recipes that meet my needs and still are enjoyed by everyone
Top of Head	I'm glad I have found some clarity

 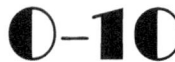 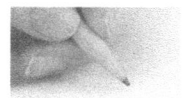

Tapping Exercise:

Think about someone you know that is overweight. What negative thoughts do you have about them? Tap while reviewing those thoughts.

I am afraid to step on a scale.

The Setup

Even though I'm afraid to step on a scale, I deeply and completely love and accept myself. Even though I'm afraid to see how much I weigh right now, I know that the scale isn't really going to tell me anything I don't already know. I choose to love and accept myself, no matter what the scale says.

The Tapping

Eyebrow	I see the scale as the enemy
Side of Eye	Sometimes I see my body as the enemy too
Under the Eye	Neither one of those views is particularly helpful for me
Nose	I'm afraid to step on the scale
Chin	Let me say it again, I'm afraid to step on the scale
Collarbone	I'M AFRAID TO STEP ON THE SCALE (louder)
Under the Arm	That seems pretty silly
Top of Head	I get the same information from the fit of my clothes and my image in the mirror

KEEP GOING TO NEXT PAGE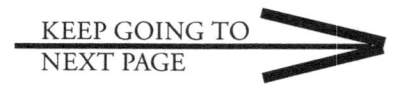

Eyebrow	I'm not fooling anyone else, and I'm not fooling myself
Side of Eye	I can step on the scale and have the number
Under the Eye	I might not like what it tells me
Nose	But it is information that I can use to motivate me
Chin	It is also information that I can use to measure my success
Collarbone	The scale is a tool that I can choose to use - or not use
Under the Arm	The choice is totally mine
Top of Head	I can choose to weigh, or not weigh. In either case, I can choose to love and accept myself while I am on this path to improved health and wellness

 **0-10**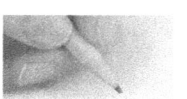

"It is no measure of health to be well adjusted to a
profoundly sick society." - Jiddu Krishnamurth

147

Nothing calms me down better than food.

The Setup

Nothing calms me down better than food. Whenever I get upset I turn to food. It always works for me. Even though nothing calms me down better than food, I don't like what it does to my body. I am open to learning new ways of calming down. I am also open to learning more about the things that upset me so that I don't even need to use food to calm myself.

The Tapping

Eyebrow	When I get upset, nothing calms me down better than food
Side of Eye	When I get upset, nothing calms me down better than food
Under the Eye	When I get upset, nothing calms me down better than food
Nose	When I get upset, nothing calms me down better than food
Chin	When I get upset, nothing calms me down better than food
Collarbone	When I get upset, nothing calms me down better than food
Under the Arm	When I get upset, nothing calms me down better than food
Top of Head	When I get upset, nothing calms be down better than food

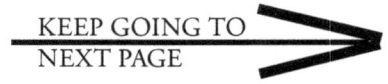

KEEP GOING TO
NEXT PAGE

Eyebrow	Food calms me down
Side of Eye	But it also is making me fat
Under the Eye	Food calms me down
Nose	And I often need to calm down
Chin	I get upset pretty often
Collarbone	And I use food to calm me down
Under the Arm	It is quick, easy, and painless
Top of Head	Well, maybe not painless

 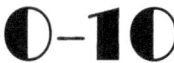 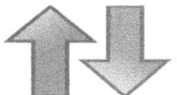

Eyebrow	Being overweight is definitely painful
Side of Eye	It is painful physically and emotionally
Under the Eye	I probably need to learn new ways to deal with my emotions
Nose	Food is quick, but the side effects last a long time
Chin	I can learn to manage my stress another way
Collarbone	I can learn to calm myself another way
Under the Arm	Even though I have used food to calm myself in the past
Top of Head	I am excited about the possibility of learning a new way

 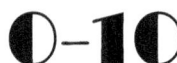 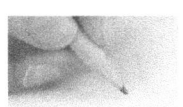

I'm too tired to work out today.

The Setup

Even though I am too tired to work out today, I love and accept myself anyway. Even though I'm too tired to work out today, I choose to love myself completely. Even though I think I'm too tired to work out today, I am open to a change of heart.

The Tapping

Eyebrow	I am too tired to work out today
Side of Eye	Just the thought of working out seems overwhelming
Under the Eye	I know I'll feel better if I at least exercise a little bit
Nose	I know I'll be less discouraged if I work out too
Chin	But I'm just too tired
Collarbone	Do I really know how I will feel later?
Under the Arm	No, not really
Top of Head	I just know I'm too tired to work out right now

KEEP GOING TO NEXT PAGE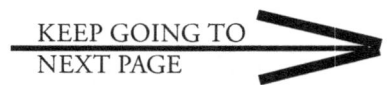

Eyebrow	I may feel a lot better after a while
Side of Eye	I choose to do some things now that could help me feel better later
Under the Eye	Then working out might not seem so overwhelming
Nose	Nobody else decides what exercise I will do
Chin	I'm the one who decides how, and how long
Collarbone	I might be able to find something that fits with my energy level
Under the Arm	I choose to keep my overall health and happiness as top priority
Top of Head	I am too tired to work out right now, but I choose to re-evaluate a little later

   0-10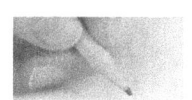

"Never before has there been such an objectively and repeatedly reliable method for freeing ourselves from fears and other negative emotions, as well as inner obstacles to health, happiness, peace, love and the manifestation of our goals in life." - Rober Elias Najemy

149

I can't believe I gained weight again.

The Setup

I just can't believe that I gained weight again. I worked so hard to lose it last time. Even though I have gained weight again, I choose to love and respect myself anyway. Even though it is difficult to believe that I am at this place again, I love myself and accept that this is a struggle for me. Even though I have gained weight again, I choose to love and accept myself.

The Tapping

Eyebrow	I've gained weight
Side of Eye	I swore it would never happen again
Under the Eye	But it did
Nose	Not only do I feel bad about my weight
Chin	But I also feel bad about my failure to keep it off
Collarbone	This makes me feel pretty stuck
Under the Arm	I worked so hard to lose the weight
Top of Head	And I don't want to face all of that hard work again

KEEP GOING TO NEXT PAGE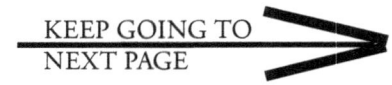

Eyebrow	I do know that I can lose the weight
Side of Eye	And knowing that does feel good
Under the Eye	Last time I wasn't even sure that I could do it
Nose	Now I know I can
Chin	Maybe it will be easier this time
Collarbone	I really don't have to make it so hard
Under the Arm	I could choose to make this fun and exciting
Top of Head	I am open to the possibility of effortless success

 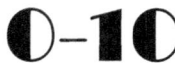 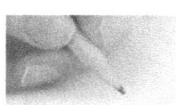

Tapping Exercise:

Before going to sleep tonight, spend at least 5 minutes tapping.

Only chocolate will make me feel better.

The Setup

I need chocolate. Only chocolate will make me feel better. I'm so upset right now. I have to eat chocolate to feel better. Even though I need chocolate right now, I deeply and completely love and accept myself.

The Tapping

Eyebrow	I need chocolate
Side of Eye	I can't stand how I am feeling
Under the Eye	And I need it to go away right now
Nose	Chocolate always works
Chin	And I have a new brownie recipe to try
Collarbone	I want to make them now
Under the Arm	But even if I make them now
Top of Head	I have to wait for them to bake

KEEP GOING TO NEXT PAGE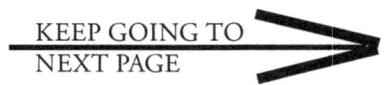

Eyebrow	Then I have to wait for them to cool
Side of Eye	I guess I will have to deal with my feelings no matter what
Under the Eye	If I use the chocolate to feel better
Nose	I will have to deal with the feelings
Chin	And with the disappointment of eating something that I know is bad for me right now
Collarbone	I don't need chocolate
Under the Arm	I need to feel better
Top of Head	There are many ways to achieve that

 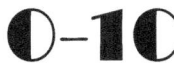 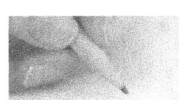

"Don't dig your grave with your own knife and fork." - English Proverb

My thoughts about food are really crazy.

The Setup

My thoughts about food are really crazy. I don't think they are normal. Even though I feel this way, I love and accept myself and all of my crazy thoughts about food. Even though I have crazy thoughts about food, I am open to learning more about this. Even though I have crazy thoughts about food, I choose to remain calm and focused about my goals.

The Tapping

Eyebrow	These crazy thoughts about food
Side of Eye	These crazy thoughts about food
Under the Eye	These crazy thoughts about food
Nose	These crazy thoughts about food
Chin	These crazy thoughts about food
Collarbone	These crazy thoughts about food
Under the Arm	These crazy thoughts about food
Top of Head	These crazy thoughts about food

   **0-10**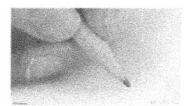

152

I feel unattractive.

The Setup

Even though I feel unattractive, I love and accept myself. Even though I feel unattractive, I am open to feeling better about myself sometime in the future. Even though I feel unattractive, I choose to treat myself with love and respect.

The Tapping

Eyebrow	I feel unattractive
Side of Eye	I feel unattractive
Under the Eye	I feel unattractive
Nose	I feel unattractive
Chin	I feel unattractive
Collarbone	I feel unattractive
Under the Arm	I feel unattractive
Top of Head	I feel unattractive

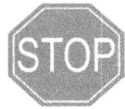   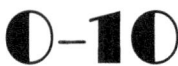   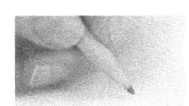

153

I don't want to exercise.

The Setup

Even though I don't want to exercise, I choose to accept myself completely. Even though I don't want to exercise, I choose to love myself completely. Even though I don't want to exercise, I choose to love and accept myself anyway.

The Tapping

Eyebrow	I don't want to exercise
Side of Eye	And I don't even know why
Under the Eye	I know I will feel better if I do
Nose	I don't want to exercise
Chin	But I will feel better physically if I do
Collarbone	I don't want to exercise
Under the Arm	But I will feel better mentally if I do
Top of Head	I don't want to exercise

KEEP GOING TO
NEXT PAGE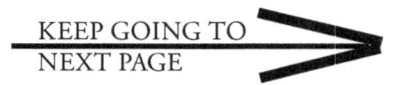

Eyebrow	But I will feel better about myself if I do
Side of Eye	I don't want to exercise
Under the Eye	But I choose to exercise anyway
Nose	I don't feel like exercising
Chin	But I can follow my plan
Collarbone	I don't feel like exercising
Under the Arm	But I do feel like being healthy
Top of Head	I can overcome this challenge to my exercise plan

   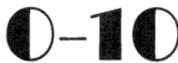   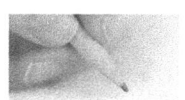

"A diet is the penalty we pay for exceeding
the feed limit." - Author Unknown

154

Vegetables just aren't fun.

The Setup

Even though I think that vegetables just aren't fun, I choose to remain open to a new way of thinking about them. Even though I think that vegetables just aren't fun, I choose to believe that there is a new way of thinking about them. Even though I think that vegetables just aren't fun, I choose to love and accept myself anyway.

The Tapping

Eyebrow	Vegetables just aren't fun
Side of Eye	That's why I don't want to eat them
Under the Eye	Everyone knows that vegetables are boring
Nose	Well, maybe not everybody
Chin	I'm told that some people really like vegetables
Collarbone	I see pictures of vegetable plates that are very pretty
Under the Arm	But those pictures don't really make me want to eat them
Top of Head	I really do wish that I liked vegetables more than I do

KEEP GOING TO
NEXT PAGE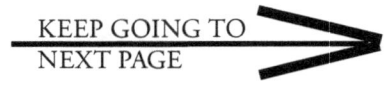

Eyebrow	I am proud of my efforts to eat more vegetables
Side of Eye	I am confident that I will be healthier
Under the Eye	When I can learn to enjoy more vegetables
Nose	Until then, I choose to be excited about learning to cook more vegetables
Chin	Until then, I choose to be excited about trying to eat more vegetables
Collarbone	I choose to look forward to a day where I'll choose vegetables over other foods
Under the Arm	It's hard to imagine
Top of Head	But I choose to move forward with excitement and confidence

 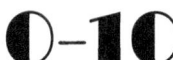 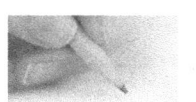

"In the Middle Ages, they had guillotines, stretch racks, whips and chains. Nowadays, we have a much more effective torture device called the bathroom scale." - Stephen Phillips

I know I'm not hungry, but I want to eat.

The Setup

Even though I want to eat, I choose to eat only when I am hungry. Even though I want to eat, I choose to eat based on my plan and not my feelings. Even though I want to eat, I love and accept myself completely.

The Tapping

Eyebrow	I really want to eat
Side of Eye	This feeling is very strong
Under the Eye	All I can think about is food
Nose	I could probably name almost everything in the refrigerator right now
Chin	I know I'm not really hungry because the fruits and vegetables aren't calling to me
Collarbone	It's the starchy and sugary stuff that I am really thinking about
Under the Arm	Instead of labeling this feeling as hunger
Top of Head	I choose to look for what this is really about

KEEP GOING TO NEXT PAGE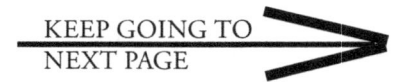

Eyebrow	The truth is that I am extremely tired
Side of Eye	It has been a stressful day
Under the Eye	I want to stay up a little while longer to watch a TV show I've been waiting to see
Nose	In the past I've used food to give me an evergy lift and keep me awake
Chin	I choose to use a different strategy tonight
Collarbone	Eating when I am tired isn't the best solution
Under the Arm	I have many choices
Top of Head	I am excited about my insight and how it leads to better solutions

 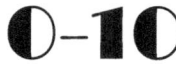 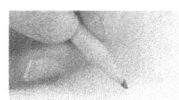

Tapping Exercise:

Begin tapping. Remember a time when you intentionally ate more food than your body needed. Recall all of the details about what was happening before you ate, during the time you were eating, and after.

I'm eating more sweets than my body can handle.

The Setup

I've been eating more sweets lately than my body can handle. It is not a good thing for my blood sugar, my weight, or my brain either. All of those things are important to me. Probably the worst thing is that it isn't good for my self esteem. I choose to love and forgive myself for this overindulgence. Even though I have been overeating with sugary foods and snacks, I choose to become more aware of my reasons for doing this. Even though it has always been hard to resist sugary foods in the past, I choose to move forward easily and confidently.

The Tapping

Eyebrow	I'm eating more sweets than my body can handle
Side of Eye	That is upsetting to me on many different levels
Under the Eye	I love the way sweet things taste
Nose	But I feel bad almost immediately after eating them
Chin	I don't like the long-term consequences either
Collarbone	I say that my health is important to me
Under the Arm	But my behavior sure doesn't show it
Top of Head	I don't think I really am aware of what I'm doing most of the time

KEEP GOING TO
NEXT PAGE →

Eyebrow	I just seem to prefer sugary foods
Side of Eye	But I hope to retrain my taste buds
Under the Eye	I want to learn to love healthy foods
Nose	That's a good way to love myself
Chin	Eating sweet things has been hard to resist
Collarbone	But I choose to move toward a healthier way of eating
Under the Arm	I choose to stop hurting myself with food
Top of Head	I am confident in my ability to eat in a more mindful and healthy way

 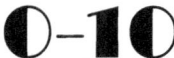 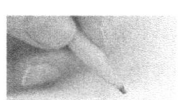

"Gluttony is an emotional escape, a sign something
is eating us." - Peter De Vries

He said my butt was big, and it really hurt.

The Setup

During my teenage years a very mean boy told me my butt was really big. His exact words were, "it is so big that it curls up in my face." Looking back now I know it was a stupid thing for him to say, but at the time it was devastating. I know that it couldn't even have been true. I wore a size 5. There is no way my butt could have been big. Even though I know that he was just being mean, and even though I let him get to me back then, and even though I have carried this emotional pain with me for decades, I choose to let it go. I choose to love and accept myself fully and unconditionally.

The Tapping

Eyebrow	He said my butt was big
Side of Eye	He really hurt my feelings
Under the Eye	I have been carrying this pain around with me for many years
Nose	I can see him as he is saying it
Chin	I can hear his voice
Collarbone	I still remember his name
Under the Arm	He was a mean little boy
Top of Head	But his words really hurt me

KEEP GOING TO NEXT PAGE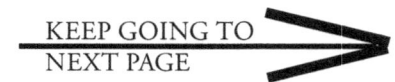

Eyebrow	Those words changed my view of myself
Side of Eye	Those words changed my view of my body
Under the Eye	I wonder how much they have impacted my weight issues
Nose	He said my butt was too big
Chin	It really wasn't big back then, but it is now
Collarbone	I choose to release the old pain on an emotional level
Under the Arm	I choose to release the trauma on an emotional level
Top of Head	I choose to release the old pain and trauma on a physical level

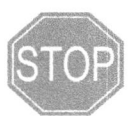 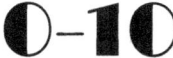 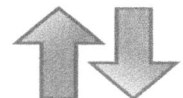

Eyebrow	Even though he said my butt was big
Side of Eye	I choose to forgive him for his cruelty
Under the Eye	Even though he said my butt was big I choose to forgive him for his immaturity
Nose	Even though he said my butt was big
Chin	I choose to forgive myself for believing him
Collarbone	Even though I have carried this old pain and trauma with me for all of these years
Under the Arm	I choose to love and respect myself now
Top of Head	I choose to love and respect myself now

 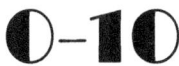 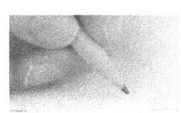

Being fat is a family trait.

The Setup

All of the women in my family have been heavy. It has gone on for generations. On an emotional level, I think I use being fat as a way of being connected. It gives me a sense of belonging to my family's heritage. Now that I am aware of this, I choose to reconsider whether this is the way I want to be connected or not. I acknowledge my desire to fit in. I acknowledge my desire to be connected. I choose to love and accept myself totally and unconditionally in spite of any poor health choices I may have made in the past.

The Tapping

Eyebrow	I'm fat
Side of Eye	My mother has been fat
Under the Eye	My grandmother was fat
Nose	My great grandmother was fat
Chin	I have aunts that were fat
Collarbone	Cousins too
Under the Arm	Most of the women in my family have been fat
Top of the Head	And now I'm carrying on this family tradition

KEEP GOING TO NEXT PAGE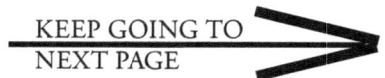

Eyebrow	I wonder if there is more to it than that?
Side of Eye	The other side of my family doesn't seem to have that trait
Under the Eye	But that is a side of the family I don't really want to relate to
Nose	I don't like to think of myself as being "like them"
Chin	Being fat could be a way of rejecting that family
Collarbone	And belong to the other family
Under the Arm	There has to be a better way to get my emotional needs met
Top of Head	I choose to find better ways to get my emotional needs met

   **0-10**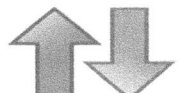

Eyebrow	I release my need to be fat in order to belong
Side of Eye	I release my need to reject affiliation with certain family members
Under the Eye	I choose to love myself enough to take care of my body
Nose	I choose to love myself enough
Chin	To make healthy emotional choices
Collarbone	I am open to clarity about this issue
Under the Arm	I am open to forgiveness
Top of Head	I am open to healing

      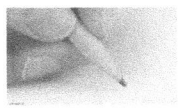

159

I can't seem to stop eating.

The Setup

Even though I can't seem to stop eating, I choose to love and accept myself anyway. Even though I can't seem to stop eating, I choose to focus on my strengths more than my weaknesses. Even though I can't seem to stop eating, I choose to keep trying and never give up on my health.

The Tapping

Eyebrow	I can't seem to stop eating
Side of Eye	I keep eating even when I'm not hungry
Under the Eye	I keep eating even when the food makes me sick
Nose	I keep eating when no one is watching
Chin	I keep eating even when there are people around
Collarbone	I can't seem to stop eating
Under the Arm	I can't seem to stop eating
Top of Head	I can't seem to stop eating

KEEP GOING TO NEXT PAGE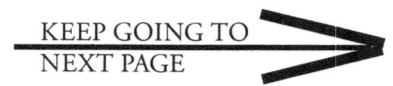

Eyebrow	It seems that I have no control over this
Side of Eye	I don't like that
Under the Eye	I am a person who wants to be in control
Nose	But if I were in control, I would be able to stop eating
Chin	I can't seem to stop eating
Collarbone	I want to learn to stop
Under the Arm	I AM learning how to stop
Top of Head	I am a work in progress

 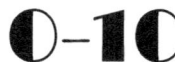 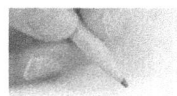

Tapping Exercise:

Think about dessert. How often do you feel the desire for dessert? Do you always give in? Why or why not? Tap while considering your answers.

I'm so mad at myself.

The Setup

Even though I am so mad at myself, I want to love and accept myself anyway. Even though I am so mad at myself, I choose to see this as a temporary situation, rather than one that is permanent. Even though I am so mad at myself, I choose to handle the situation with self-respect and self-love.

The Tapping

Eyebrow	I am so mad at myself right now
Side of Eye	And I choose to deal with the problem calmly
Under the Eye	I am so mad at myself right now
Nose	And I choose to treat myself respectfully
Chin	I am so mad at myself right now
Collarbone	I choose to love myself anyway
Under the Arm	I am so mad at myself right now
Top of Head	But I choose not to be self-destructive with food

 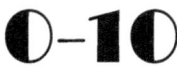 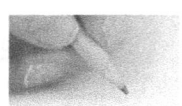

161

I have a weird relationship with food.

The Setup

I have a weird relationship with food. It isn't just food to me. It means so much more than that. Even though I have this weird relationship with food, I am open to getting to the bottom of it. Even though I have a weird relationship with food, I am excited to know that even this can change. Even though I have a weird relationship with food, I choose to love and accept myself unconditionally.

The Tapping

Eyebrow	Weird relationship with food
Side of Eye	Weird relationship with food
Under the Eye	Weird relationship with food
Nose	Weird relationship with food
Chin	Weird relationship with food
Collarbone	Weird relationship with food
Under the Arm	Weird relationship with food
Top of Head	Weird relationship with food

 **0–10**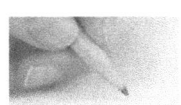

I don't understand why I keep eating like this.

The Setup

I don't understand why I keep eating like this. I know better. My head is totally behind a new diet plan. Something keeps getting in my way. I keep getting in my way. It is so frustrating. Even though I keep eating like this, I choose to love and accept myself just as I am. Even though I'm frustrated with my eating habits, I choose to do things differently in the future. Even though I keep getting in my own way, I choose to reclaim my power.

The Tapping

Eyebrow	I keep blowing it
Side of Eye	I have the best intentions
Under the Eye	But that only lasts about 5 minutes
Nose	Then I'm just out of control
Chin	This pattern keeps repeating
Collarbone	And it is so frustrating to me
Under the Arm	I don't understand why I keep getting in the way of myself
Top of Head	I certainly know what I need to eat and what I don't

KEEP GOING TO NEXT PAGE
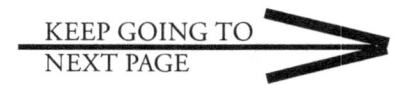

Eyebrow	Nobody is making me eat the foods that are bad for me
Side of Eye	I do the shopping
Under the Eye	Nobody is making me buy those things either
Nose	There must be something else going on here
Chin	I am open to clarity about this issue
Collarbone	I don't seem to be completely in control of my eating
Under the Arm	Not what I eat
Top of Head	And not how much I eat

 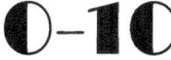 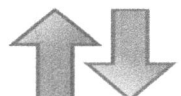

Eyebrow	But I choose to remember that this can change
Side of Eye	I am frustrated by my eating habits
Under the Eye	But I choose to remember that this can change
Nose	I keep getting in my own way
Chin	But I choose to remember that this can change
Collarbone	I don't like the way I have been eating
Under the Arm	But I choose to remember that this can change
Top of Head	I choose to remember that I am a work in progress

 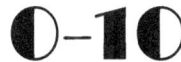 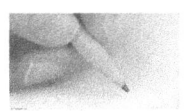

I am fat.

The Setup

I am fat. That word really stings. Everybody knows that fat is bad. Saying that I am fat is the same thing as saying that I am bad. It also brings up all kinds of beliefs and prejudices that I don't really want to admit that I have, and I really don't want to apply them to myself. Who am I kidding? Saying that I am fat floods me with self-loathing. Even though I am full of self-loathing because I am fat, I choose to remember that my body can change. Even though I am full of self-loathing because I am fat, I choose to remember that my viewpoint can change. Even though I am full of self-loathing because I am fat, I choose to remember that my feelings can change.

The Tapping

Eyebrow	I am fat
Side of Eye	And I don't like that fact
Under the Eye	I am fat
Nose	And that makes me feel like a bad person
Chin	I am fat
Collarbone	And that makes me dislike myself
Under the Arm	I am fat
Top of Head	And that makes me loathe myself.

KEEP GOING TO NEXT PAGE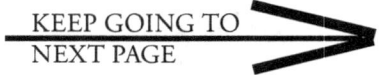

Eyebrow	I am full of self loathing
Side of Eye	I loathe my body because of how fat I am
Under the Eye	I loathe myself because of how fat I am
Nose	I choose to remember that this can be a temporary situation
Chin	It is simply the status of my body right now
Collarbone	My body is only one aspect of me
Under the Arm	I am fat
Top of Head	But I choose to love myself no matter what

 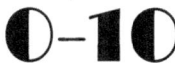 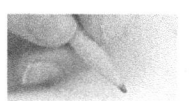

"In general, mankind, since the improvement of cookery, eats twice as much as nature requires." - Benjamin Franklin

Cookies make me lose control.

The Setup

Even though cookies make me lose control, I deeply and completely love and accept myself anyway. Even though cookies make me lose control, and I can't seem to enjoy just one of them without eating them all, I love and accept myself anyway. Even though cookies make me lose control and I always significantly overeat whenever they are available, I love and accept myself anyway.

The Tapping

Eyebrow	Cookies make me lose control
Side of Eye	I lose control whenever cookies are around
Under the Eye	I can't eat just one
Nose	I can't even eat just two
Chin	I can't relax until they are all gone
Collarbone	I always intend to exercise self control
Under the Arm	But I don't have any self control when there are cookies available
Top of Head	Cookies make me lose control

KEEP GOING TO NEXT PAGE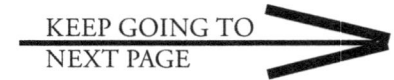

Eyebrow	I don't like feeling out of control
Side of Eye	And I certainly don't like giving up my control to a plate full of cookies
Under the Eye	Big cookies, little cookies, soft cookies, crisp cookies
Nose	They all make me lose control
Chin	Just one cookie sets off the cravings
Collarbone	Out of control about cookies
Under the Arm	I feel out of control about cookies
Top of Head	Losing control about cookies

 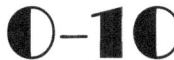 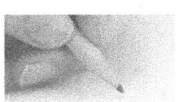

"Those who think they have not time for bodily exercise will
sooner or later have to find time for illness." - Edward Stanley

165

I'm not good enough the way I am now.

The Setup

I don't feel like I am good enough the way I am now. I believe that I have to be thin to be good enough. I feel like I have to be thin to be worthy. I know that I am not good enough and therefore unworthy the way my body is now. My rational brain says that this isn't true and that I am good enough just the way I am and that I will still be good enough if I lose weight or gain weight, but that doesn't change how I feel on the inside. Even though I feel like I am not good enough the way I am now, I am open to learning to love myself just a little bit more. Even though I don't feel like I am good enough the way I am right now, I choose to act on my rational thoughts anyway.

The Tapping

Eyebrow	I hate how I look
Side of Eye	I'm not good enough
Under the Eye	I hate how I look
Nose	I'm not good enough
Chin	I hate how I look
Collarbone	I'm not good enough
Under the Arm	I hate how I look
Top of Head	I'm not good enough

KEEP GOING TO NEXT PAGE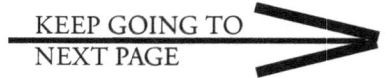

Eyebrow	I hate how I look
Side of Eye	I'm not good enough
Under the Eye	Not the way I am right now
Nose	I'm not good enough
Chin	How I look proves that
Collarbone	I'm not good enough
Under the Arm	I hate how I look
Top of Head	I'm not good enough

 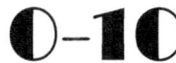 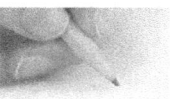

Tapping Exercise:

Begin tapping. Imagine walking up to an unlimited buffet table, loaded with all of your favorite foods. Spend a few minutes tapping about the thoughts and feelings that arise. Now, imagine what the best response would be. How would you like to feel when finding yourself in that situation? What would some good options be? Spend a few minutes tapping while visualizing yourself making those good choices.

166

I don't know what to wear.

The Setup

I don't know what to wear. Nothing looks good on this body. Everything stylish is made for thin women, not women with hips. I don't know what to wear. I want to look good but I don't know how. Even though I am confused about what to wear, I am open to clarity. Even though I don't like the way I look in most of my clothing, I am open to finding options. Even though I don't know what to wear, I am open to loving myself anyway.

The Tapping

Eyebrow	What should I wear?
Side of Eye	I just don't know
Under the Eye	My hips are too big
Nose	My clothes don't fit right
Chin	I am so confused
Collarbone	I don't know what to do
Under the Arm	I really want to look attractive
Top of Head	I don't know what to wear

KEEP GOING TO NEXT PAGE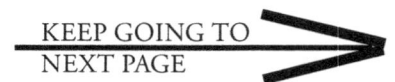

Eyebrow	All of these feelings about clothing
Side of Eye	Nothing looks good on me right now
Under the Eye	And I find that very upsetting
Nose	Upset about clothing
Chin	I'm so upset about clothing
Collarbone	These feelings about clothing
Under the Arm	I have all of these feelings about clothing
Top of Head	I'm upset about my clothing

 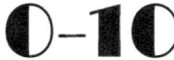 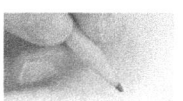

"Lack of activity destroys the good condition of
every human being, while movement and methodical
physical exercise save it and preserve it." - Plato

Bring on the pizza.

The Setup

I am craving pizza. I can almost taste it. I want thick crust, gooey cheese, and lots of pepperoni. I know that isn't a healthy meal for me, but I want it anyway. Even though I am having this strong craving for pizza, I love and accept myself completely. Even though I have this craving for pizza, I deeply and completely love and accept myself. Even though I am having this strong craving, I love and accept myself anyway.

The Tapping

Eyebrow	This pizza craving
Side of Eye	I am craving pizza
Under the Eye	I am craving cheese
Nose	I am craving crust
Chin	I am craving pepperoni
Collarbone	This pizza craving
Under the Arm	This strong pizza craving
Top of Head	This pizza craving

   **0-10**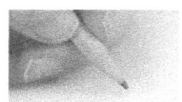

I want a snack, but I'm not really hungry.

The Setup

Even though I am craving a snack right now, I acknowledge that I'm not really hungry. I just want one. I think I'm probably bored. I've been sitting for a long time. Other people around me are snacking, and I want to be snacking too. I have carrots with me to munch on, but that's not really what I want. My brain is looking for some sugar excitement. Even though I want a sugary snack right now, I am open to more clarity about this issue. Even though I want a sugary snack right now, I choose to love and accept myself whether I eat one or not.

The Tapping

Eyebrow	I want a snack
Side of Eye	I'm not really hungry
Under the Eye	But I really want a snack
Nose	This snack craving
Chin	I want a snack now
Collarbone	This craving for a snack
Under the Arm	I want a snack
Top of Head	This intense craving

   **0–10**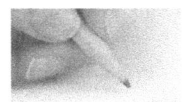

169

I made more bad food choices.

The Setup

I made more bad food choices. I worry about what is happening to my body. I worry about what is happening to my health. I worry about what other people would think if they knew. I feel ashamed of my food choices. I should have better control than that. My feelings about this are very strong. I feel shame to the core of my being. I made more bad food choices - AGAIN!

The Tapping

Eyebrow	These bad food choices
Side of Eye	Bad food choices
Under the Eye	I made more bad food choices
Nose	All of these bad food choices
Chin	I made bad food choices again
Collarbone	I am ashamed of my bad food choices
Under the Arm	This shame about my choices
Top of Head	This guilt about my choices

KEEP GOING TO NEXT PAGE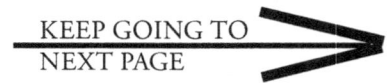

Eyebrow	These bad food choices
Side of Eye	I am embarrassed about my bad food choices
Under the Eye	I am afraid of what others will think of me
Nose	I am afraid for my health
Chin	I made more bad food choices
Collarbone	These bad food choices
Under the Arm	I hate these bad food choices
Top of Head	I want to stop making bad food choices

 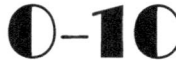 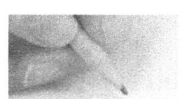

"A sad soul can kill you quicker than a germ." - John Steinbeck

I have no idea what to make for dinner and that is always dangerous.

The Setup

Even though I don't know what to make for dinner, and that is always dangerous, I love and accept myself anyway. Even though I don't know what to make for dinner and I didn't make a plan ahead of time, I love and accept myself anyway. Even though I have no idea what I am going to make for dinner and that increases the likelihood that I will stray from my overall diet plan, I love and accept myself anyway, no matter what.

The Tapping

Eyebrow	I don't know what to make for dinner
Side of Eye	That has caused problems for me in the past
Under the Eye	I'm feeling anxious
Nose	Because I know what can happen
Chin	I didn't plan ahead
Collarbone	That is a setup for disaster
Under the Arm	At least it has been in the past
Top of Head	I didn't make a plan for dinner

KEEP GOING TO NEXT PAGE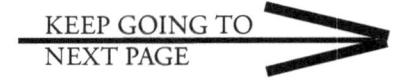

Eyebrow	And now I have to come up with something
Side of Eye	I'm feeling anxious
Under the Eye	This anxiety about making dinner
Nose	This anxiety about making dinner
Chin	This anxiety about making dinner
Collarbone	This anxiety about making good choices for dinner
Under the Arm	This anxiety about making good choices for dinner
Top of Head	This anxiety about making good choices for dinner

 **0-10**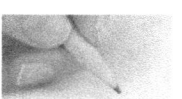

"The root of all health is in the brain. The trunk of it is in emotion. The branches and leaves are the body. The flower of health blooms when all parts work together." - Kurdish Saying

I would love to be an intuitive eater.

The Setup

I've read articles about being an intuitive eater. Frankly they tick me off. If I had any ability to do that, I would. Reading an article like that makes me want to eat more. Even though I am having strong feelings in response to this topic, I choose to seek clarity. Even though I am having strong feelings in response to this topic, I choose to seek peace. Even though I am having strong feelings in response to this topic, I choose to seek health.

The Tapping

Eyebrow	I'm not an intuitive eater
Side of Eye	And I want to be
Under the Eye	It ticks me off that I'm not
Nose	I'm not sure I really believe that anyone is
Chin	That seems like such a foreign concept
Collarbone	Actually, I'm jealous
Under the Arm	I want it to be easy
Top of Head	And for me its not

KEEP GOING TO NEXT PAGE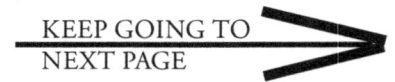

Eyebrow	I'm having a strong reaction to this
Side of Eye	I feel anger
Under the Eye	I feel resentment
Nose	I feel jealousy
Chin	Those are strong emotions for something that seems so trivial
Collarbone	I am open to clarity about these feelings
Under the Arm	I am open to loving myself even with these feelings
Top of Head	I am open to a change in my perception

 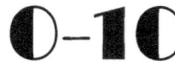 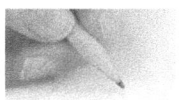

Tapping Exercise:

Spend 10 minutes tapping through the points. Notice which ones feel the best.

When I am bored I want to eat.

The Setup

Even though I want to eat because I am bored, I deeply and completely love and accept myself. Even though I am bored and that makes me want to eat, I love and accept myself and these feelings. Even though I am bored and I want to eat, I love and accept myself.

The Tapping

Eyebrow	I am bored and I want to eat
Side of Eye	I am bored and I want to eat
Under the Eye	This boredom
Nose	I want to eat
Chin	I want to eat because of the boredom
Collarbone	I am bored and want to eat
Under the Arm	I am bored
Top of Head	I want to eat

KEEP GOING TO NEXT PAGE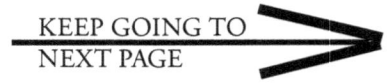

Eyebrow	This boredom
Side of Eye	I really want to eat
Under the Eye	I am so bored
Nose	I want to eat because I'm bored
Chin	I am so bored
Collarbone	I want to eat
Under the Arm	I want to eat to make the boredom go away
Top of Head	I don't want to be bored

 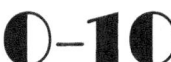 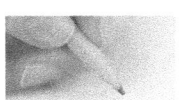

"Everyone should be his own physician. We ought to assist and not force nature. Eat with moderation what agrees with your constitution. Nothing is good for the body but what we can digest. What medicine can produce digestion? Exercise. What will recruit strength? Sleep. What will alleviate incurable ills? Patience." - Voltaire

My diet plan fell apart.

The Setup

Even though my diet plan fell apart, I love and respect myself. Even though my diet plan fell apart, which means I ate things that I wish I hadn't, I choose to remember that I can get back on track any time I want to. Even though my diet plan fell apart again, I am open to loving myself completely in spite of my struggles.

The Tapping

Eyebrow	My diet plan fell apart
Side of Eye	I ate things that I wish I hadn't
Under the Eye	I feel bad about my diet errors
Nose	I feel like a failure when I don't follow the plan
Chin	When my plan falls apart I feel like giving up
Collarbone	My diet plan fell apart again
Under the Arm	This isn't the first time
Top of Head	Unfortunately, it probably isn't the last time either

KEEP GOING TO
NEXT PAGE
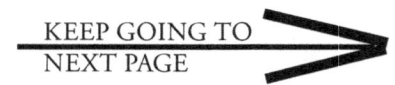

Eyebrow	I am open to learning more about why my plans fall apart
Side of Eye	My diet plan fell apart this time
Under the Eye	But I can get back on track when I want to
Nose	My diet plan fell apart
Chin	But that doesn't mean I have to fail
Collarbone	My diet plan failed again
Under the Arm	But this could be an opportunity to learn more about myself
Top of Head	I choose to remain open to success

 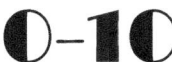 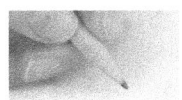

"I am convinced that unconditional love is the most powerful known stimulant of the immune system. If I told patients to raise their blood levels of immune globulins or killer T cells, no one would know how. But if I can teach them to love themselves and others fully, the same changes happen automatically. The truth is: love heals." - Bernie Siegel

Getting old means getting fat.

The Setup

Even though I have old programming that says that getting old means that it is inevitable that you get fat, I deeply and completely accept myself. Even though I have old programming about age and weight, I am open to any evidence, for or against this belief. Even though I have thought that getting old means that you have to get fat, I am open to clarity.

The Tapping

Eyebrow	Getting old means getting fat
Side of Eye	Getting old means getting fat
Under the Eye	Getting old means getting fat
Nose	Getting old means getting fat
Chin	Getting old means getting fat
Collarbone	Getting old means getting fat
Under the Arm	Getting old means getting fat
Top of Head	Getting old means getting fat

   **0-10**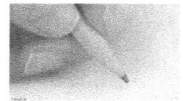

I am angry about my weight.

The Setup

Even though I am angry about my weight, I am choosing to love and accept myself just as I am right now. It isn't easy. I'm struggling with how to separate what I weigh from who I am. In spite of this struggle, I choose to love myself and treat myself with love and dignity.

The Tapping

Eyebrow	I am angry about my weight
Side of Eye	I don't like it at all
Under the Eye	I acknowledge that being angry isn't likely to help much
Nose	And it won't help at all if I take that anger out on myself
Chin	I am angry about my weight
Collarbone	This anger about my weight
Under the Arm	I have this anger about my weight
Top of Head	I am open to a more loving frame of mind

0-10

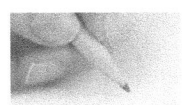

176

I just ate a whole box of cookies.

The Setup

Even though I just ate a whole box of cookies, I choose to look forward to the day when I can control my eating better. Even though I just ate a whole box of cookies, I am open to learning more about why I did it. Even though I just ate a whole box of cookies, I am hopeful that I can do better in the future.

The Tapping

Eyebrow	I just ate a whole box of cookies
Side of Eye	That was more than a whole day's calories
Under the Eye	I ate more calories than my body needs
Nose	It was a lot of sugar
Chin	They contained a lot of fat too
Collarbone	The first one tasted good
Under the Arm	Actually, the second one tasted good too
Top of Head	After that it was really just mindless eating

KEEP GOING TO NEXT PAGE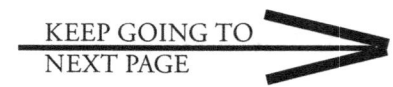

Eyebrow	I know why I ate them
Side of Eye	I was upset
Under the Eye	The sugar worked for a while
Nose	But then I felt bad
Chin	Because I did something that was unhealthy for me
Collarbone	It didn't solve the problem
Under the Arm	And it didn't help me avoid the conflict
Top of Head	I choose to learn from this mistake

 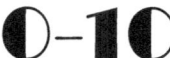 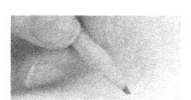

"You can learn to follow the inner self, the inner physician that tells you where to go. Healing is simply attempting to do more of those things that bring joy and fewer of those things that bring pain." - O. Carl Simonton

Healthy eating takes too much planning.

The Setup

Even though healthy eating seems to take too much planning for me, I am open to new ways of thinking about this. Even though I would like eating to be a little more spontaneous sometimes, I deeply and completely love and accept myself. Even though healthy eating seems to take more planning than I want, I choose to look for ways to make things easier in the future.

The Tapping

Eyebrow	Healthy eating takes too much planning
Side of Eye	That makes eating healthy foods much too difficult for me
Under the Eye	I want it to be easy
Nose	I want it to be quick
Chin	I want eating to be spontaneous
Collarbone	I get tired of planning everything I eat
Under the Arm	It would be nice to think about what I want
Top of Head	Instead of what I need

KEEP GOING TO NEXT PAGE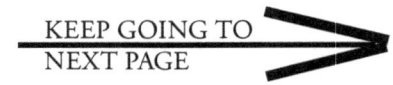

Eyebrow	But that doesn't change how I feel about it
Side of Eye	I don't want to do so much planning
Under the Eye	I suspect that there are many ways to make the planning easier
Nose	I know there are ways to build more spontaneity into my meals
Chin	I could have several healthy options available
Collarbone	And then choose the one I want on a whim
Under the Arm	That would still require some planning
Top of Head	But not every day

   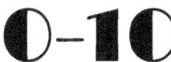   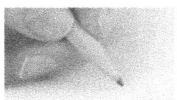

Tapping Exercise:

Begin tapping. Remember a time when you were a child and were coerced or forced to eat a food you didn't like.

178

I hate to drink plain water.

The Setup

I know water is good for me. I know I'm supposed to drink lots of it everyday. Unfortunately, I just don't like to drink water. Even though I hate to drink plain water, I acknowledge that my body needs it. Even though I hate to drink plain water, I love and accept myself. Even though I hate to drink plain water, I choose to remain open to all of my options.

The Tapping

Eyebrow	I hate to drink plain water
Side of Eye	It just doesn't taste good
Under the Eye	That is not really a fair statement
Nose	Most of the time it doesn't taste like anything
Chin	Maybe I object to its nothingness
Collarbone	I hate drinking plain water
Under the Arm	I don't do it very often
Top of Head	And that isn't good for my body or my brain

KEEP GOING TO NEXT PAGE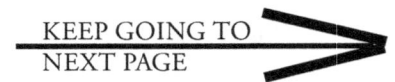

Eyebrow	I would like to think differently about this
Side of Eye	I would like to drink more water so that my body can be healthy
Under the Eye	Avoiding water is nothing more than a bad habit
Nose	I have overcome other bad habits
Chin	I am sure I can overcome this one too
Collarbone	Even though I have avoided drinking plain water in the past
Under the Arm	I am choosing to remain open to new possibilities in the future
Top of Head	I am looking forward to the day when I crave water more

 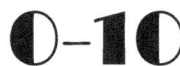 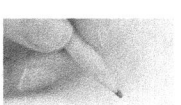

"Every day we touch what is wrong, and, as a result, we are becoming less and less healthy. That is why we have to learn to practice touching what is not wrong—inside us and around us. When we get in touch with our eyes, our heart, our liver, our breathing, and our non-toothache and really enjoy them, we see that the conditions for peace and happiness are already present." - Thich Nhat Hanh

My metabolism isn't cooperating with me.

The Setup

I have a sluggish metabolism. It just isn't cooperating with my desire to lose weight easily. It feels like a constant battle and that battle is wearing me down. Even though I have a sluggish metabolism, I choose to love and accept myself just the way I am right now. Even though I would really like to lose weight, and I want it to be a bit easier, I choose to love and accept myself whether it is easy or hard.

The Tapping

Eyebrow	This sluggish metabolism
Side of Eye	I have a sluggish metabolism
Under the Eye	And I blame my metabolism for all of my problems
Nose	All of my problems are because of my metabolism
Chin	If my metabolism was faster
Collarbone	I could lose weight faster
Under the Arm	I would be happier faster too

KEEP GOING TO
NEXT PAGE
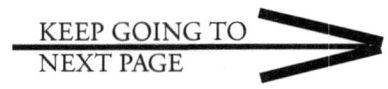

Eyebrow	My metabolism is sluggish
Side of Eye	And I'm doing battle with it
Under the Eye	But that makes me fighting against myself
Nose	That feels like I am hating a part of me
Chin	That can't be a good thing
Collarbone	I want to love myself, even my metabolism
Under the Arm	My metabolism is a part of me
Top of Head	And I choose to love it

 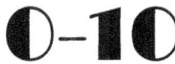 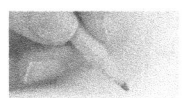

"I have come to understand that some of the deepest and most effective healing is not found at a doctor's office or a hospital, but rather from inside ourselves. Our bodies are designed for self-healing, and we are capable of both boosting and blocking that ability." - Dr. Daju Suzanne Friedman

When I think diet, I think deprivation.

The Setup

My very first thought when I think about dieting is deprivation. No more of the foods I love and crave. With that as a first thought it is no wonder that I am having trouble really committing to a healthy diet program. I'm not sure how to get that reaction out of my head. It has been that way for as long as I remember. I do want to think about healthy eating without feeling deprivation, but I just don't really believe it can be true. I choose to be open to a change in my thinking. I choose to be open to a change in my feelings. I choose to be open to a change of heart.

The Tapping

Eyebrow	Dieting means deprivation to me
Side of Eye	No more cookies
Under the Eye	No more ice cream
Nose	No more cake
Chin	No more potato chips
Collarbone	No more chocolate
Under the Arm	Why would I want that?
Top of Head	I am hoping it can be different

KEEP GOING TO NEXT PAGE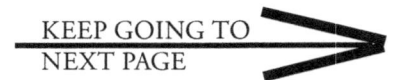

Eyebrow	But I'm not feeling all that certain
Side of Eye	I am open to feeling less deprivation
Under the Eye	And more joy in being healthy
Nose	Although dieting has meant deprivation to me in the past
Chin	I am learning to love and accept myself anyway
Collarbone	I have always associated diet with deprivation
Under the Arm	But I believe that can change
Top of Head	I choose to let go of deprivation

 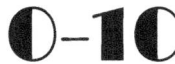 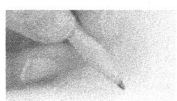

Tapping Exercise:

How many situps or crunches do you believe that you can do? Go ahead and do some. Did you make the number you predicted? Now spend some time tapping while visualizing yourself doing 10 more. After tapping, give it a try.

181

I hate it that they can eat and I can't.

The Setup

I feel incredibly jealous that other people can eat, but I can't eat. What I really mean is that other people seem to be able to eat whatever they want, but if I do that I gain weight. It's just not fair. This jealousy isn't a good thing and I know that, but it is really how I feel. I am very jealous. I'm angry that I can't eat whatever I want and if I can't do it, I don't want anyone to be able to do it. I accept my feelings about this. I accept my thoughts about this. I accept myself and my beliefs about this.

The Tapping

Eyebrow	They can eat whatever they want
Side of Eye	And I can't
Under the Eye	I hate that
Nose	I'm very jealous
Chin	And I feel like whining
Collarbone	In reality I am whining
Under the Arm	This jealousy about food
Top of Head	This jealousy about dieting

KEEP GOING TO NEXT PAGE
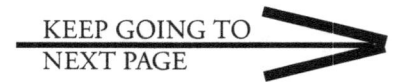

Eyebrow	This jealousy about weight loss
Side of Eye	I want things to be as easy for me
Under the Eye	As it looks like it is for others
Nose	I'm whining again
Chin	I am jealous and I know it
Collarbone	I am jealous and I accept myself
Under the Arm	I am jealous and I accept myself
Top of Head	I accept myself and my feelings

 **0-10**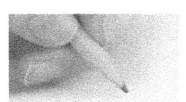

"Body and soul cannot be separated for purposes of treatment, for they are one and indivisible. Sick minds must be healed as well as sick bodies." - C. Jeff Miller

182

I hate how I look.

The Setup

Even though I hate how I look, I choose to love myself anyway. Even though I hate how I look, I choose to accept myself anyway. Even though I hate how I look, I choose to love and accept myself anyway.

The Tapping

Eyebrow	I hate how I look
Side of Eye	I hate how I look
Under the Eye	I hate how I look
Nose	I hate how I look
Chin	I hate how I look
Collarbone	I hate how I look
Under the Arm	I hate how I look
Top of Head	I hate how I look

KEEP GOING TO
NEXT PAGE
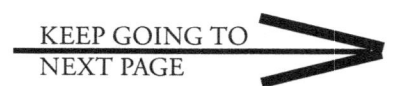

Eyebrow	I choose to focus on the things I do love
Side of Eye	I choose to treat myself with kindness
Under the Eye	I choose to move forward with my life
Nose	I choose to act respectfully toward my body
Chin	I choose to be gentle
Collarbone	I choose to see myself as beautiful
Under the Arm	I choose to see myself as attractive
Top of Head	I choose to see myself as confident

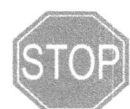 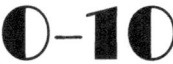 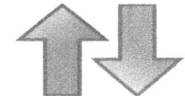

Eyebrow	I hate how I look
Side of Eye	But I choose to focus on the things I do love
Under the Eye	I hate how I look
Nose	I choose to treat myself with kindness
Chin	I hate how I look
Collarbone	But I choose to move forward with my life
Under the Arm	I hate how I look
Top of Head	I choose to see myself as beautiful, attractive, and confident

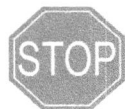 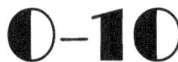 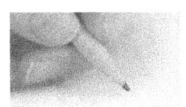

183

If I eat a little bit I spiral out of control.

The Setup

Even though I spiral out of control if I eat a little bit of some foods, I choose to remain optimistic that I can regain balance. Even though I have spiraled out of control in the past when I have eaten even a little bit of some foods, I love and accept myself anyway. Even though I have been out of control with my eating, I am open to learning new ways of living and eating.

The Tapping

Eyebrow	I'm afraid of some foods
Side of Eye	Because I spiral out of control if I eat them
Under the Eye	I don't like being afraid of food
Nose	And I don't like being afraid of my reaction to it
Chin	I know that there may be a chemical issue that makes some foods act like a drug in my brain
Collarbone	I know there are emotional reasons that some foods get to me too
Under the Arm	I don't like that out of control feeling
Top of Head	It really scares me to think that I have such little control over my own thoughts, feelings, and behaviors

KEEP GOING TO NEXT PAGE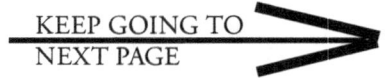

Eyebrow	I really can't eat just one when it comes to some foods
Side of Eye	I'm really better off to not have those foods anywhere near me
Under the Eye	But that makes me sad
Nose	I feel angry too
Chin	Angry at myself
Collarbone	Angry at the food
Under the Arm	And angry at everyone else that can eat just a little bit
Top of Head	I acknowledge that my feelings are okay

 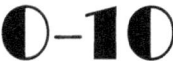 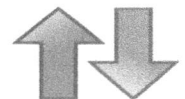

Eyebrow	I choose to treat myself more tenderly
Side of Eye	I choose to love myself in spite of this challenge
Under the Eye	I know I have choices
Nose	And with tapping I have options
Chin	This may not be as hard as I seem to be making it
Collarbone	I am looking forward to a time when this will seem easy
Under the Arm	I choose to rebalance my brain and body in healthy ways
Top of Head	I choose to focus on what I can control rather than what I can't

 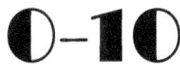 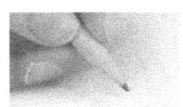

184

Nobody really likes exercise.

The Setup

I don't think anyone really enjoys exercise. I know I certainly don't. So much of my time is spent working. Why would I want to do something I don't enjoy during my free time? I don't believe anyone really enjoys exercise. Even though I have this limiting belief, I love and accept myself. Even though I have this belief that keeps me from being as fit and healthy as I could be, I love and accept myself. Even though I have this belief that sounds more like an excuse than rational thought, I love and accept myself.

The Tapping

Eyebrow	Nobody really likes exercise
Side of Eye	Nobody really likes exercise
Under the Eye	Nobody really likes exercise
Nose	Nobody really likes exercise
Chin	Nobody really likes exercise
Collarbone	Nobody really likes exercise
Under the Arm	Nobody really likes exercise
Top of Head	Nobody really likes exercise

0-10

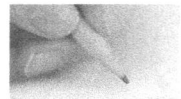

Isn't food supposed to be fun?

The Setup

Even though I believe that food is supposed to be fun, and feel that right now it isn't fun for me, I deeply and completely love and accept myself. Even though I want food to be more fun than it is right now, I love and accept myself anyway. Even though food isn't as fun as I would like it to be right now, I am open to seeing this in a new way.

The Tapping

Eyebrow	I want food to be more fun
Side of Eye	Food isn't as fun as I would like it to be
Under the Eye	Fun food doesn't seem to fit with with a diet plan
Nose	I want to have more fun with food
Chin	But I don't want to gain weight
Collarbone	I'm really frustrated right now
Under the Arm	And I don't like my choices
Top of Head	I want food to be more fun

   **0-10**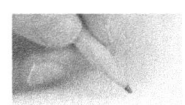

I don't know how to be normal.

The Setup

I don't feel normal when I think about eating, food, dieting, and exercise. I don't know how to be normal. Nothing about this feels normal to me. I have a strong need to feel normal, even though I don't know what that is. I am open to clarity. I am open to acceptance. I am open to change. Even though I don't think I know how to be normal, I choose to love and accept myself anyway.

The Tapping

Eyebrow	Don't know how to be normal
Side of Eye	Don't know how to be normal
Under the Eye	Don't know how to be normal
Nose	Don't know how to be normal
Chin	Don't know how to be normal
Collarbone	Don't know how to be normal
Under the Arm	Don't know how to be normal
Top of Head	Don't know how to be normal

KEEP GOING TO NEXT PAGE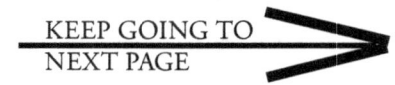

Eyebrow	Don't know how to be normal
Side of Eye	But I choose to be open to change
Under the Eye	Don't know how to be normal
Nose	But I choose to seek clarity
Chin	Don't know how to be normal
Collarbone	But I love myself anyway
Under the Arm	Don't know how to be normal
Top of Head	But I choose to feel calm while exploring this issue

   0-10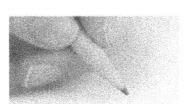

"Chronic disease is a foodborne illness. We ate our way into this mess, and we must eat our way out." - Mark Hyman

187

I hate my flabby thighs.

The Setup

Even though I hate my flabby thighs, I am trying to love and accept myself anyway.
Even though I hate my flabby thighs, I would like to learn to love myself completely.
Even though I hate my flabby thighs, I choose to treat myself lovingly.

The Tapping

Eyebrow	I really hate my flabby thighs
Side of Eye	They jiggle when I walk
Under the Eye	They are very unattractive
Nose	I can't remember a time when I had beautiful thighs
Chin	They rub together
Collarbone	They are really ugly
Under the Arm	I don't like to look at them
Top of Head	I don't want anyone else to see them either

KEEP GOING TO
NEXT PAGE

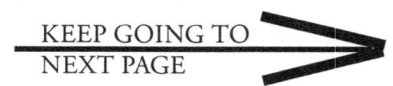

Eyebrow	I hate my flabby thighs
Side of Eye	I hate the front of them
Under the Eye	I hate the back of them
Nose	I hate the sides too
Chin	I hate my flabby thighs
Collarbone	My thighs are disgusting
Under the Arm	They are dimpled and ugly
Top of Head	I hate flabby thighs

 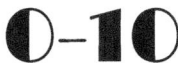 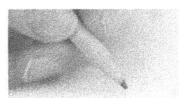

"The more you eat, the less flavor; the less you
eat, the more flavor." - Chinese Proverb

My brain is lying to me right now.

The Setup

Even though my brain is lying to me right now and telling me I'm hungry, I choose to remember that I ate a short while ago and this is just a misperception. Even though my brain is lying to me right now and telling me that I should eat, I choose to remember my health goals. Even though my brain is telling me I'm hungry, I know that this cannot be the truth and I choose not to eat based on a lie.

The Tapping

Eyebrow	I can't sleep because I'm hungry
Side of Eye	I want to get up out of bed and get a snack
Under the Eye	That will help me sleep
Nose	No one can fall asleep when they are hungry
Chin	Certainly not me
Collarbone	But I know I'm not really hungry
Under the Arm	I ate a healthy meal a few hours ago
Top of Head	My body got everything it needed

KEEP GOING TO NEXT PAGE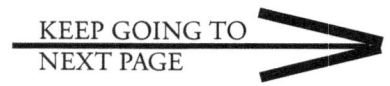

Eyebrow	What I'm feeling right now isn't really hunger
Side of Eye	That's just what my brain is calling it
Under the Eye	I probably am tired, frustrated, angry, lonely, sad, or uncomfortable
Nose	Food won't fix any of those things
Chin	In fact, eating more food than my body needs will only make them worse
Collarbone	I choose to eat based on facts, not lies
Under the Arm	Even though I am convinced that I am hungry right now
Top of Head	I choose to love and accept myself just as I am

 **0-10**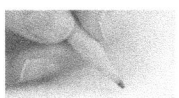

Tapping Exercise:

Is it true that you cannot eat just one? Pick any food that you believe you will not be able to stop after eating just one. Place it in front of you. Really look at it. Smell it. Taste it. Then start tapping. After several minutes, take one bite. Tap again. Take another bite. Keep tapping until you are confident that you can walk away.

Cooking new things makes me anxious.

The Setup

Even though cooking new things makes me anxious, I am excited about the possibility of success. Even though cooking new things makes me anxious, I love and accept all of my thoughts and feelings. Even though cooking new things makes me worried and anxious, I choose to remember that I've been successful many times before.

The Tapping

Eyebrow	Cooking new things makes me anxious
Side of Eye	I get worried about how it will turn out
Under the Eye	I also get worried about looking foolish
Nose	And feeling incompetent
Chin	The nervousness starts when I buy the new ingredients
Collarbone	It continues until I taste what I have cooked
Under the Arm	Cooking new things often makes me anxious
Top of Head	That anxiety often reaches a pretty high level

KEEP GOING TO NEXT PAGE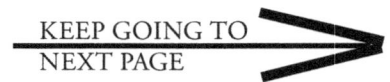

Eyebrow	Sometimes I even chicken out and end up throwing food away without preparing it
Side of Eye	I don't want to do that anymore
Under the Eye	I've been pretty successful recently with my cooking
Nose	Things aren't always perfect, but I'm getting better
Chin	I've purchased, prepared, and eaten things that I have never tried before
Collarbone	And I've liked them
Under the Arm	My anxiety is really unfounded
Top of Head	I choose to be excited about new cooking possibilities

STOP **0–10**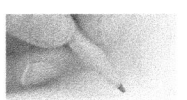

"Physical fitness is not only one of the most important keys to a healthy body, it is the basis of dynamic and creative intellectual activity - John F. Kennedy

190

If I had someone to cook for me I could do it.

The Setup

Even though I don't believe that I can do this by myself, I deeply and completely love and accept myself. I feel like I need someone to cook for me in order to be successful. I don't believe in my own ability to do what needs to be done. In spite of my disbelief, I choose to love and accept myself.

The Tapping

Eyebrow	If I only had someone to cook for me, I could maintain a healthy weight and healthy body
Side of Eye	At least that is what I tell myself
Under the Eye	Rather than acknowledge my own choices and behaviors
Nose	I am looking for something outside of myself to blame
Chin	Not only could I avoid responsibility
Collarbone	I could avoid having to take an action
Under the Arm	I can just sit down, give up, and continue gaining weight
Top of Head	Why am I so willing to give up?

KEEP GOING TO NEXT PAGE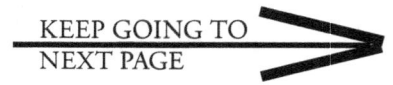

Eyebrow	Is it true that I would be more successful with someone else doing the cooking?
Side of Eye	Probably not
Under the Eye	Maybe what I need is someone to plan my meals
Nose	Perhaps I lack the creativity
Chin	Probably not. I bet I could plan someone else's menu
Collarbone	Blaming my problem on something outside of me isn't the answer
Under the Arm	I have trouble changing my self-destructive behavior
Top of Head	I probably should tap on that

 **0-10**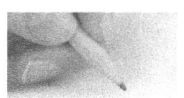

"It is health that is real wealth and not pieces of gold and silver." - Mahatma Gandhi

I gained it back so quickly.

The Setup

Even though I am upset with myself because I gained it back so quickly, I am open to clarity about this issue. Even though I am upset with myself because I gained it back so quickly, I choose to be gentle with myself right now. Even though I am upset with myself because I gained it back so quickly, I am open to learning about what happened.

The Tapping

Eyebrow	I gained it back so quickly
Side of Eye	I gained it back so quickly
Under the Eye	That is very upsetting to me
Nose	I can't believe that this has happened
Chin	I gained it back so quickly
Collarbone	This feels devastating to me
Under the Arm	I gained it back so quickly
Top of Head	I feel like I have failed

KEEP GOING TO NEXT PAGE
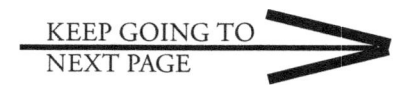

Eyebrow	No, I feel like a failure
Side of Eye	I gained it back so quickly
Under the Eye	I am so upset by this
Nose	I gained it back so quickly
Chin	I feel very bad about this
Collarbone	I feel pretty bad about me
Under the Arm	I gained it back so quickly and I feel awful
Top of Head	I gained it back so quickly

 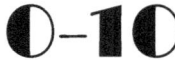 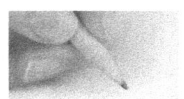

"Leave all the afternoon for exercise and recreation, which are as necessary as reading. I will rather say more necessary because health is worth more than learning." - Thomas Jefferson

I am embarrassed about how I look.

The Setup

I am so embarrassed about how I look. When I look at myself in the mirror I cringe. I worry about what other people think when they see how out of shape my body is. I am so embarrassed. I feel ashamed. Other people must have negative feelings about me too. In spite of this, I love and accept myself completely.

The Tapping

Eyebrow	I am embarrassed about how I look
Side of Eye	I am embarrassed about my weight
Under the Eye	I am embarrassed about how my clothes fit
Nose	I am embarrassed about my flabby arms
Chin	I am embarrassed about my sagging skin
Collarbone	I am embarrassed about my lack of muscles
Under the Arm	I am embarrassed about my terrible complexion
Top of Head	I am embarrassed about how I look

KEEP GOING TO NEXT PAGE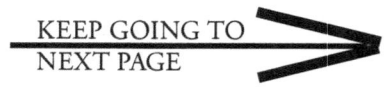

Eyebrow	If I could just manage my weight, everything would be better
Side of Eye	Well, maybe not everything
Under the Eye	But it would sure help
Nose	I am embarrassed about how I look
Chin	But I'm also embarrassed because how I look says a lot about me
Collarbone	That is probably the real reason I'm embarrassed
Under the Arm	How I look is a reflection of my self control
Top of Head	I am embarrassed by my appearance and my lack of self control

 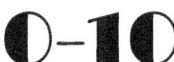 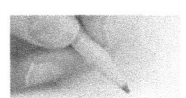

"If we get our self-esteem from superficial places, from our popularity, appearance, business success, financial situation, health, any of these, we will be disappointed, because no one can guarantee that we'll have them tomorrow." - Kathy Ireland

Eating healthy is boring.

The Setup

Even though eating healthy is very boring, I choose to remember my goals. Even though eating healthy is very boring, I choose to remember my health. Even though healthy food is boring, I love and accept myself and all of my feelings about this.

The Tapping

Eyebrow	Eating healthy is boring
Side of Eye	Healthy food is boring
Under the Eye	I am open to a change of opinion
Nose	Eating healthy is boring
Chin	Healthy food is boring
Collarbone	I am open to a change of heart
Under the Arm	Eating healthy is boring
Top of Head	Healthy food is boring

KEEP GOING TO NEXT PAGE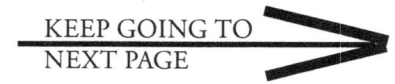

Eyebrow	I am open to new feelings about this
Side of Eye	Eating healthy is boring
Under the Eye	Healthy food is boring
Nose	I am open to finding ways to make my healthy food more interesting
Chin	Eating healthy is boring
Collarbone	Healthy food is boring
Under the Arm	But maybe that doesn't have to be true
Top of Head	I choose to remain open to the possibilities

 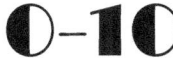 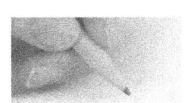

"Boredom: the desire for desires." - Leo Tolstoy

I hate looking at myself in the mirror.

The Setup

Even though I hate looking in the mirror, I love and accept myself anyway. Even though looking in the mirror at myself is disgusting to me, I love and accept myself anyway. Even though I hate looking at myself in the mirror, I choose to love and accept myself anyway.

The Tapping

Eyebrow	I hate looking at myself in the mirror
Side of Eye	I hate looking at myself in the mirror
Under the Eye	I hate looking at myself in the mirror
Nose	I hate looking at myself in the mirror
Chin	I hate looking at myself in the mirror
Collarbone	I hate looking at myself in the mirror
Under the Arm	I hate looking at myself in the mirror
Top of Head	I hate looking at myself in the mirror

   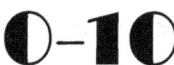   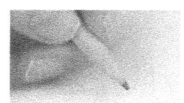

I'm jealous of skinny people.

The Setup

Even though I am jealous of skinny people, I choose to love and accept myself just as I am. Even though I am jealous of skinny people, I choose to let go of this jealousy. Even though I feel jealous of skinny people, and imagine that they are somehow better than I am, I choose to love and accept myself.

The Tapping

Eyebrow	I am jealous of skinny people
Side of Eye	I want to be skinny too
Under the Eye	This irrational jealousy
Nose	Jealous of skinny people
Chin	This jealousy
Collarbone	I'm so jealous
Under the Arm	I am jealous of skinny people
Top of Head	This jealousy

   **0-10**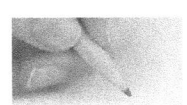

I want to be admired for who I am, not what I look like.

The Setup

I have an image in my head that suggests that I can be more certain of people's intentions if I am fat than if I am thin. My rational brain says that this is probably not true, but it feels true. Even though I have this irrational belief, I choose to be open to a new way of thinking about things. Even though I have this irrational belief, and I suspect it is getting in the way of my health, I love and accept myself anyway. Even though I have this irrational belief, I accept all of my thoughts and feelings.

The Tapping

Eyebrow	I want to be admired
Side of Eye	I am afraid that I won't know how people really feel
Under the Eye	If I am thin and attractive
Nose	If I am fat and someone admires me
Chin	I can know that it is really about me, not my appearance
Collarbone	I am suspicious of the motives of others
Under the Arm	I use my fat to protect myself
Top of Head	I don't trust myself to know what people really want from me

KEEP GOING TO
NEXT PAGE
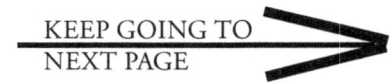

Eyebrow	I choose to trust my own instincts
Side of Eye	I choose to focus on my physical health
Under the Eye	I am worthy of respect
Nose	I care a lot about what others think of me
Chin	Now I choose to care about what I think of me
Collarbone	I am able to overcome my irrational thoughts
Under the Arm	I believe in myself
Top of Head	I choose to love and respect myself

 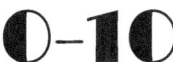 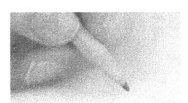

"When you are content to be simply yourself and don't compare
or compete, everybody will respect you." - Lao Tzu

My cravings always win.

The Setup

Even though it seems like my cravings always win, I deeply and completely love and accept myself anyway. Even though it seems like my cravings always win, I choose to continue to try. My cravings are a part of me, and I accept myself.

The Tapping

Eyebrow	My cravings always win
Side of Eye	So it doesn't seem worth it to even try
Under the Eye	I might as well just go ahead and eat it
Nose	If I fight it and then lose, I just end up feeling worse
Chin	Even though it seems that my cravings always win
Collarbone	I know that it isn't really true
Under the Arm	Sometimes I am able to resist
Top of Head	I am open to learning about what makes me more successful at one time

KEEP GOING TO NEXT PAGE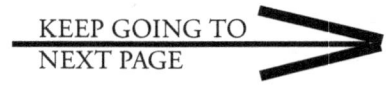

Eyebrow	And less successful at another
Side of Eye	My cravings don't always win
Under the Eye	My cravings sometimes win
Nose	In reality, my cravings aren't against me
Chin	They are a part of me
Collarbone	My cravings are a signal that something needs my attention
Under the Arm	I can choose to deal with it without food
Top of Head	I can choose to continue toward my goals

 **0–10**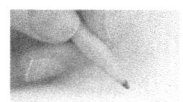

Tapping Exercise:

Do you remember the self-discovery exercises at the beginning of this book? You were asked to write down what the downside is for you in changing your weight. Begin tapping about the first answer. When you are done, cross it off of the list and move on the next one.

I am confused by the contradictory advice out there about diets.

The Setup

There seems to be so much contradictory information out there about diets and food. That confuses me. Sometimes it makes me feel trapped. Other times I'm just overwhelmed and don't do anything at all. Even though I'm confused, I am open to clarity. Even though I often feel overwhelmed about it all, I choose to believe that I can find a way that is right for me. Even though I sometimes get stuck and don't do anything at all, I can love and accept myself just as I am.

The Tapping

Eyebrow	There is so much information out there about diets
Side of Eye	Most of it doesn't agree
Under the Eye	You can find a diet that says almost anything
Nose	All of that information is very confusing
Chin	All of my confusion sometimes makes me not want to do anything
Collarbone	Do I eat vegan?
Under the Arm	Do I eat low carb?
Top of Head	Should I fast?

KEEP GOING TO NEXT PAGE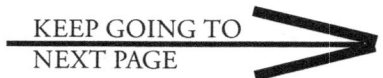

Eyebrow	Do I eat more frequently?
Side of Eye	Who knows? And that makes me confused and frustrated
Under the Eye	I choose to take action for my health
Nose	My body knows what I need
Chin	All I have to do is listen
Collarbone	I can choose to eat in a way that nourishes my body
Under the Arm	I can choose to eat in a way that nourishes my soul
Top of Head	I don't have to follow anyone else's diet. I can follow mine

 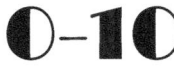 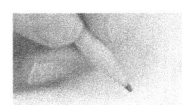

Tapping Exercise:

Browse back through some of the tapping scripts that you have worked on. As you re-read them, reflect upon how your thoughts and feelings have changed in regard to the topic. If your intensity has gone back up, or if there is a new aspect that has emerged, be sure to tap again.

199

Once I mess up it is hard to get back on track.

The Setup

Even though it is hard to get back on track once I mess up, I deeply and completely love and accept myself. Even though it is really hard to get back on track once I mess up with my eating, I choose to learn from the situation and love myself anyway. Even though it is hard, almost impossible, for me to get back on track after I mess up, I love and accept myself, in spite of my struggles.

The Tapping

Eyebrow	It is hard to get back on track once I mess up
Side of Eye	It is hard to get back on track once I mess up
Under the Eye	It is hard to get back on track once I mess up
Nose	It is hard to get back on track once I mess up
Chin	It is hard to get back on track once I mess up
Collarbone	It is hard to get back on track once I mess up
Under the Arm	It is hard to get back on track once I mess up
Top of Head	It is hard to get back on track once I mess up

KEEP GOING TO NEXT PAGE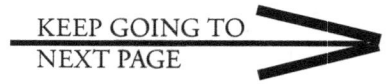

Eyebrow	In fact, sometimes it is so hard that I don't get back on track for days
Side of Eye	Then I feel bad about myself
Under the Eye	And it takes even longer to get back on track
Nose	I seem to focus on the difficulty, rather than the end goal
Chin	I want it to be easier
Collarbone	I want it to be effortless
Under the Arm	I know that is unrealistic
Top of Head	But it probably doesn't have to be as difficult as I am making it

 **0-10**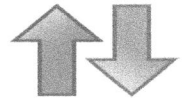

Eyebrow	I could choose to focus on my success
Side of Eye	I could even challenge myself to see how quickly I can get back on track
Under the Eye	That would give me more excuses to celebrate
Nose	I usually feel great about my successes
Chin	I can keep that in mind
Collarbone	GBOT - Get back on track
Under the Arm	That's my new motto
Top of Head	GBOT!

 **0-10**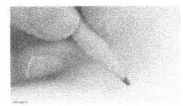

I am afraid to get on the scale.

The Setup

I am afraid to get on the scale. It is going to tell me something I already know, but somehow it seems more real when I see the actual number. Even though I am afraid to get on the scale, I love and accept myself anyway. Even though I am afraid to get on the scale, I love and accept myself anyway. Even though I am afraid to get on the scale, I love and accept myself and my fear.

The Tapping

Eyebrow	Fear of the scale
Side of Eye	Fear of the scale
Under the Eye	Fear of the numbers on the scale
Nose	Fear of the scale
Chin	I don't want to face the facts
Collarbone	Without the number I can pretend everything is okay
Under the Arm	Fear of the scale
Top of Head	I am afraid to get on the scale

   **0–10**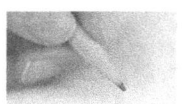

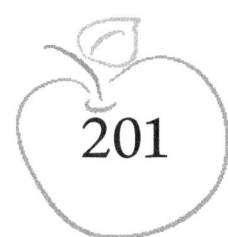

201

Situps, Pushups, and Pullups - Oh My.

The Setup

Even though I hate situps, pushups, and pullups, I choose to love and respect my body and my health. Even though I hate situps, pushups, pullups and most other forms of exercise, I choose to love and respect my body and myself. Even though I hate exercise, I choose to love and accept myself with or without it.

The Tapping

Eyebrow	I hate situps
Side of Eye	I hate pushups
Under the Eye	I hate pullups
Nose	I hate all of them
Chin	I hate situps, pushups, and pullups
Collarbone	I strongly dislike exercise
Under the Arm	Even though I hate these exercises
Top of Head	I choose to love and respect my body and my health

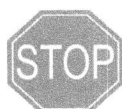 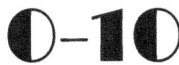 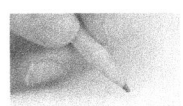

202

I just want it to be easy.

The Setup

Even though I just want it to be easy, I deeply and completely love and accept myself. Even though this whole diet thing seems to be too hard for me, I love and accept myself, including my thoughts and feelings about this. Even though I'm having a strong emotional reaction to how difficult dieting feels to me, I am open to feeling better about this.

The Tapping

Eyebrow	I just want it to be easy
Side of Eye	I want eating to be easy
Under the Eye	I want exercise to be easy
Nose	I want dieting to be easy
Chin	I want having a strong healthy body to be easy
Collarbone	It might be easy for some people
Under the Arm	And I feel like screaming and whining because it is not easy for me
Top of Head	Then I feel bad for screaming and whining like a two year old

KEEP GOING TO NEXT PAGE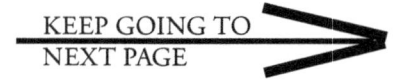

Eyebrow	That just makes me want to eat more to comfort myself
Side of Eye	I know that my reactions are "okay"
Under the Eye	But I don't like them
Nose	I know I don't have to act on these feelings
Chin	But I just don't want to have these feelings at all
Collarbone	I want it to be easy
Under the Arm	I don't want to struggle
Top of Head	IT'S NOT FAIR!

 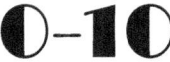 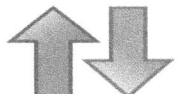

Eyebrow	IT'S NOT FAIR!
Side of Eye	Wow. That felt good to say
Under the Eye	I accept that this won't be as easy as I would like it to be
Nose	Perhaps I can look for ways to make some of it easier
Chin	And be aware of ways that I'm making some of it more difficult than it has to be
Collarbone	I don't have to go from difficult to easy all at once
Under the Arm	And I can learn to accept myself, even when I am feeling like a whiny two year old
Top of Head	Perhaps I can continue to love myself even if I'm not handling this perfectly

 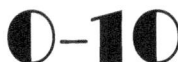 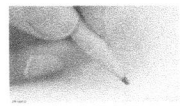

Losing weight would be easier if I lived alone.

The Setup

Even though I believe that losing weight would be easier if I lived alone, I choose to lose weight anyway. Even though it might really be easier to lose weight if I lived alone, I choose to do it whether it is easy or hard. Even though I'm feeling resentful that living with others makes my weight loss harder, I choose to look for solutions that would make my weight loss easier.

The Tapping

Eyebrow	It would be so much easier to lose weight if I lived alone
Side of Eye	All of these forbidden foods wouldn't be staring me in the face when I feel weak
Under the Eye	I could just have the things here that are good for my food plan
Nose	I guess that means I have no willpower
Chin	That isn't really true all of the time
Collarbone	But there are times when my willpower is low
Under the Arm	And at those times it probably would be easier
Top of Head	But what about loneliness?

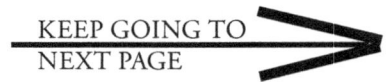

KEEP GOING TO
NEXT PAGE

Eyebrow	I eat when I'm lonely too
Side of Eye	Having people around helps me to avoid that kind of emotional eating
Under the Eye	I guess I'm just looking for excuses
Nose	That isn't going to get me where I want to go
Chin	It would be better to use other strategies
Collarbone	Instead of blaming others for my challenges
Under the Arm	I can choose to remain strong in the face of food challenges
Top of Head	I can choose to stick to my plan

 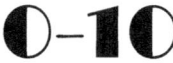 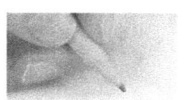

"Respect your efforts, respect yourself. Self-respect leads to self-discipline. When you have both firmly under your belt, that's real power." - Clint Eastwood

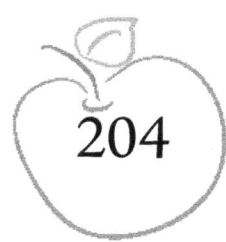

I'm so sick of being fat.

The Setup

I am so sick of being fat. I've been fat forever. It is disgusting. I'm disgusting. I am trying to love myself in spite of these thoughts and feelings. I choose to love and accept myself just as I am. Even though I'm fed up with my body size I am open to learning to love and accept myself better.

The Tapping

Eyebrow	I am so sick of being fat
Side of Eye	I hate the way I look
Under the Eye	I hate the way I feel
Nose	I hate the way my clothes fit
Chin	I hate diets
Collarbone	I hate thinking about food
Under the Arm	Sometimes I even hate me
Top of Head	I'm so sick of being fat

KEEP GOING TO NEXT PAGE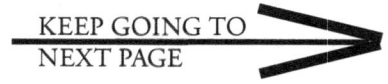

Eyebrow	Hating myself doesn't really help anything
Side of Eye	But I am really sick of this
Under the Eye	Hating my body isn't really helping anything either
Nose	But I am so sick of my struggle with weight
Chin	I'm really frustrated
Collarbone	I don't want to be overweight
Under the Arm	I want a healthier body
Top of Head	I don't want to hate myself or my body any more

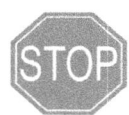 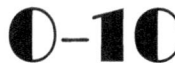 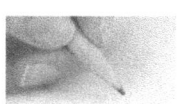

"I've come to believe that all my past failure and frustration were actually laying the foundation for the understandings that have created the new level of living I now enjoy." - Tony Robbins

205

I can't lose weight so why try?

The Setup

Even though I can't seem to lose weight and I question whether it's worth it to even try, I accept myself just where I am. Even though I can't lose weight and don't see the purpose in even trying, I am choosing to do things differently now. Even though I can't seem to lose weight and I'm considering actually giving up, I choose to love and accept myself anyway.

The Tapping

Eyebrow	I can't lose weight
Side of Eye	I've tried so many times before
Under the Eye	And I always fail
Nose	I can't lose weight
Chin	So I might as well give up
Collarbone	I don't know why I bother to even try
Under the Arm	I can't lose the weight
Top of Head	I feel like giving up

KEEP GOING TO NEXT PAGE

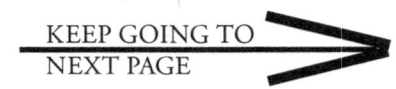

Eyebrow	The things I have tried in the past didn't work
Side of Eye	But I could choose to do things differently this time
Under the Eye	I'm not exactly sure what to do next
Nose	But I would like to feel more hopeful
Chin	I choose to reclaim my power
Collarbone	I choose to see myself in different, more loving ways
Under the Arm	I choose to love and accept myself
Top of Head	Whether I lose weight or not

 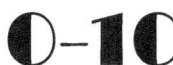 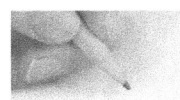

Tapping Exercise:

At the beginning of the book you were asked to rate your emotional or energetic response to some words, phrases, and statements. Rate them again now. Is there any change? Be sure to tap if any of them have increased in intensity.

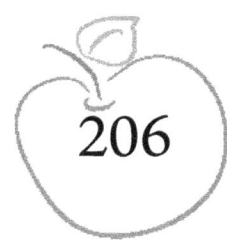

I am so tired.

The Setup

Even though I am so tired right now, I choose to believe that I will feel better soon. Even though I am so tired right now, I choose to believe that I will be okay. Even though I am so tired right now, I am open to learning what my body is trying to tell me.

The Tapping

Eyebrow	I am so very tired right now
Side of Eye	I am very tired
Under the Eye	I am so tired
Nose	So very tired
Chin	I am so tired right now
Collarbone	I can barely get moving
Under the Arm	I am so very tired
Top of Head	I am so tired right now

KEEP GOING TO NEXT PAGE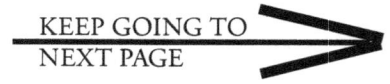

Eyebrow	But I choose to believe things will get better
Side of Eye	I am so tired right now
Under the Eye	I choose to remember that this is temporary
Nose	I am so tired right now
Chin	I am open to learning what this is about
Collarbone	My body is trying to tell me something
Under the Arm	Even though I am so tired right now
Top of Head	I am open to my body's wisdom

 **0-10**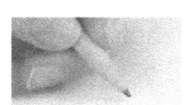

"The purpose of our lives is to be happy." -
Tenzin Gyatso, the 14th Dalai Lama

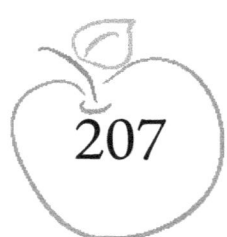

207

I really thought it would be different for me this time.

The Setup

I really thought it would be different for me this time, but it wasn't. I've struggled with my weight for so long. I guess my struggle isn't over yet. Even though I really thought it would be different for me this time, I choose to achieve my goals no matter how long it takes me. Even though I thought it would be easier this time, I choose to achieve my goals, no matter how hard it is. Even though I thought it would be different for me this time, I acknowledge my struggle and all of my feelings about it.

The Tapping

Eyebrow	I thought it would be different for me this time
Side of Eye	But this time seems to be a lot like the last time
Under the Eye	I guess that means that next time will be the same too
Nose	Since this time is the same as last time
Chin	I guess I am doomed to always be a failure
Collarbone	I feel like a failure
Under the Arm	I might as well give up
Top of Head	I don't really mean that

KEEP GOING TO NEXT PAGE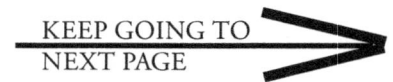

Eyebrow	I may need to change more things in order to be successful
Side of Eye	I may need to get more clear about my goals
Under the Eye	I may need more information
Nose	I may need to ask for more support
Chin	As long as I don't give up
Collarbone	I choose to believe that I can be successful
Under the Arm	I thought it would be different this time
Top of Head	And it is

 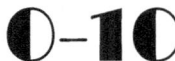 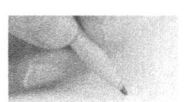

"Life is not about how fast you run or how high you climb but how well you bounce." - Vivian Komori

208

I ate chocolate chips right out of the bag.

The Setup

I stood in my kitchen and ate chocolate chips right out of the bag. I poured out handfuls of them and ate them. They were not part of my eating plan. Even though I ate the chocolate chips, I choose to forgive myself. Even though I blew my diet plan by eating the chocolate chips, I choose to forgive myself. Even though I ate the chocolate chips right out of the bag, I choose to remember that I can get back on track right now.

The Tapping

Eyebrow	I ate the chocolate chips right out of the bag
Side of Eye	I choose to forgive myself
Under the Eye	I blew my diet plan
Nose	Time to get back on track
Chin	I ate the chocolate chips
Collarbone	I forgive myself
Under the Arm	I ate chocolate chips right out of the bag
Top of Head	Time to get back on track

0-10

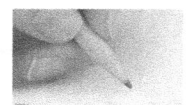

209

I don't want to be on a diet.

The Setup

Even though I am resistant to being on a diet, I accept my thoughts. Even though I am resistant to being on a diet, I accept my feelings. Even though I am resistant to being on a diet, I love and accept myself completely.

The Tapping

Eyebrow	I don't want to be on a diet
Side of Eye	I don't want to be on a diet
Under the Eye	I don't want to be on a diet
Nose	I don't want to be on a diet
Chin	I don't want to be on a diet
Collarbone	I don't want to be on a diet
Under the Arm	I don't want to be on a diet
Top of Head	I don't want to be on a diet

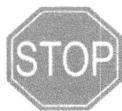   **0–10**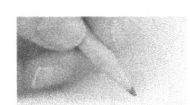

Sometimes it just feels too hard to eat the right things.

The Setup

Some days I just don't have the energy or motivation to eat the right things. I know what to do. I plan to do the right things, but then something happens to derail me. Even though it sometimes just feels too hard, I can love myself even when my motivation is weakening. Even though I sometimes believe this excuse that I'm using, I choose to love and accept myself anyway. Even though I wish eating right was easier for me, I choose to do whatever it takes to improve my health and wellbeing.

The Tapping

Eyebrow	It feels too hard
Side of Eye	It is hard to eat the right things
Under the Eye	Right now it is feeling very hard
Nose	It feels so hard
Chin	I would like to eat the right things
Collarbone	But I really want it to be easier
Under the Arm	It seems so hard
Top of Head	Too hard to eat the right things

KEEP GOING TO NEXT PAGE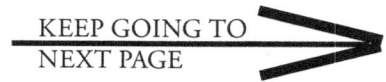

Eyebrow	Even though it seems too hard
Side of Eye	I choose to take care of myself the best I can
Under the Eye	Eating right seems too hard for me
Nose	I choose to take care of myself anyway
Chin	Sometimes it feels too hard
Collarbone	But I choose to love and accept myself anyway
Under the Arm	Eating right is too hard
Top of Head	But I trust in my ability to do this anyway

0-10

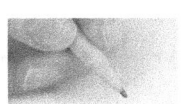

"Chronic malnutrition, or the lack of proper nutrition over time directly contributes to three times as many child deaths as food scarcity. Yet surprisingly, you don't really hear about this hidden crisis through the morning news, Twitter or headlines of major newspapers." - Cat Cora

I don't order food, I order comfort.

The Setup

When I go to a restaurant, I don't really order food I order comfort. I think about how I will feel more than how it will nourish my body. I think I would be healthier if I thought about nourishment when eating and comfort when I'm doing other things. Even though I have food and comfort somehow confused, I love and accept myself and am thankful that I am finally getting some clarity about this issue. Even though I have confused food and comfort in the past, I am excited about a new way of thinking about this. Even though I have confused food and comfort in the past, and I am feeling just a little stubborn about giving it up, I love and accept myself anyway.

The Tapping

Eyebrow	I need comfort
Side of Eye	And I do it with food
Under the Eye	I have confused food with comfort
Nose	And I would like to find a way to deal with that
Chin	I want comfort
Collarbone	I haven't been good about getting it except through food
Under the Arm	I want that to change
Top of Head	This need to get comfort through food

KEEP GOING TO NEXT PAGE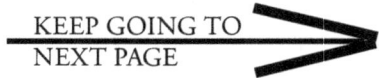

Eyebrow	I have a need to get comfort through food
Side of Eye	Even though I want comfort
Under the Eye	I choose to let food be food
Nose	It is okay to enjoy it
Chin	But it doesn't - CAN'T - fill up the empty spot inside of me
Collarbone	It is okay to want comfort
Under the Arm	It is okay to like food
Top of Head	I choose to seek other ways to get comfort in my life

 **0-10**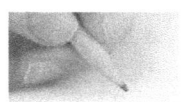

Tapping Exercise:

Begin tapping. Repeat the word "failure" aloud. Continue tapping while focusing on the thoughts and feelings associated with failure.

I hate my body.

The Setup

I hate my body, and I guess that means I hate me. That doesn't feel very good to say out loud. It doesn't feel very good to feel it on the inside either. I hate my body and unfortunately I treat my body like I hate it too. I wonder what would happen if I started to love my body. Would I treat it like I love it? Oh, I hope so. Even though I hate my body, I am open to learning to love it anyway. Even though I hate my body, I choose to begin loving myself - All of me. Even though I hate my body, I am open to loving myself anyway.

The Tapping

Eyebrow	I hate my body
Side of Eye	I have all of this hatred toward my body
Under the Eye	I hate my body
Nose	It doesn't feel good to hate my body
Chin	And it doesn't feel good to hate any part of myself
Collarbone	I do feel like I deserve it though
Under the Arm	I hate my body
Top of Head	I don't want to admit that

KEEP GOING TO NEXT PAGE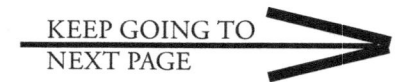

Eyebrow	But it would actually feel odd to love this body
Side of Eye	How could anyone love a body that looks like mine?
Under the Eye	I feel like I should only love a perfect body
Nose	I hate my body because it is not perfect
Chin	I guess I hate myself because I'm not perfect
Collarbone	My body is proof of that
Under the Arm	I am open to loving myself, even if I'm not perfect
Top of Head	I am also open to loving my body because it is part of me.

 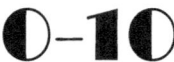 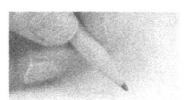

"Fitness is a curve. You can be Lance Armstrong, or you can be really out of shape at the opposite end. People enter the curve wherever they are and then they can move up the curve, by better nutrition and better exercise." - Gordon Strachan

213

I swore that I would never be this fat ever again.

The Setup

I swore that I would never be this fat ever again. Wrong. I let myself down. I am embarrassed that I couldn't keep my promise to myself. I'm angry about this failure. I'm frustrated by how ineffective I've been with my diet and exercise. In spite of all of these feelings, I choose to love and accept myself anyway.

The Tapping

Eyebrow	I swore I would never be this fat again
Side of Eye	But here I am
Under the Eye	I feel like I let myself down
Nose	I feel embarrassed that I didn't achieve my goal
Chin	I am angry with myself
Collarbone	And I feel like a failure
Under the Arm	These feelings are very disturbing to me
Top of Head	The weight is a problem

KEEP GOING TO NEXT PAGE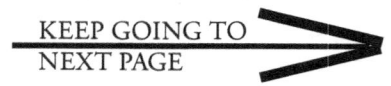

Eyebrow	But the feelings I have seem to be more of a problem right now
Side of Eye	I didn't want to gain this weight
Under the Eye	I made a vow to myself
Nose	And I really tried to keep it
Chin	I was not successful
Collarbone	That doesn't make me a failure
Under the Arm	It means I didn't succeed at this thing right now
Top of Head	I choose to love and accept myself anyway

 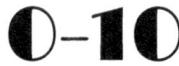 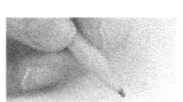

"Develop an attitude of gratitude, and give thanks for everything that happens to you, knowing that every step forward is a step toward achieving something bigger and better than your current situation." - Brian Tracy

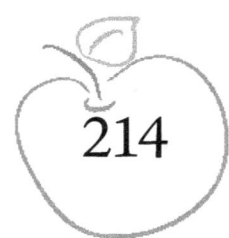

214

I don't like fish.

The Setup

Everyone says that fish is healthy, but I don't like fish. Can I still be healthy if I don't eat fish? Even though I don't like to eat fish, I choose to find other ways to be healthy and strong. Even though I don't like to eat fish, I choose to remain open to the possibility that I could find ways to eat fish that I might like. Even though I haven't learned to enjoy fish before, I love and accept myself completely.

The Tapping

Eyebrow	I don't like fish
Side of Eye	I don't like fish
Under the Eye	I don't like fish
Nose	I don't like fish
Chin	I don't like fish
Collarbone	I don't like fish
Under the Arm	I don't like fish
Top of Head	I don't like fish

0-10

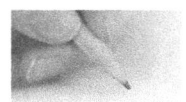

I am craving ice cream.

The Setup

Even though I am craving ice cream right now, I choose to love and respect myself enough to eat based on rational thought, not cravings or emotions. Even though I am craving ice cream right now, I choose to love and respect myself enough to eat based on rational thought, not cravings or emotions. Even though I am craving ice cream right now, I choose to love and respect myself enough to eat based on rational thought, not cravings or emotions.

The Tapping

Eyebrow	Ice cream craving
Side of Eye	I am craving ice cream
Under the Eye	This ice cream craving
Nose	Ice cream
Chin	This craving
Collarbone	Ice cream craving
Under the Arm	This intense craving
Top of Head	I am craving ice cream

   **0-10**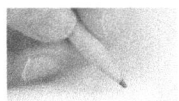

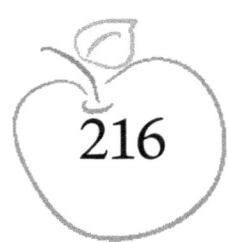

216

I have food confused with love.

The Setup

Even though I have food confused with love, I love and accept myself anyway. Even though I have food confused with love, I love and accept myself. Even though I have food confused with love, I accept my thoughts, feelings, and behaviors.

The Tapping

Eyebrow	I have food confused with love
Side of Eye	I have food confused with love
Under the Eye	I have food confused with love
Nose	I have food confused with love
Chin	I have food confused with love
Collarbone	I have food confused with love
Under the Arm	I have food confused with love
Top of Head	I have food confused with love

KEEP GOING TO
NEXT PAGE
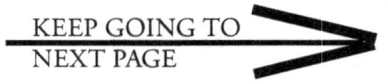

Eyebrow	This food love confusion
Side of Eye	This food love confusion
Under the Eye	This food love confusion
Nose	This food love confusion
Chin	This food love confusion
Collarbone	This food love confusion
Under the Arm	This food love confusion
Top of Head	This food love confusion

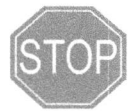 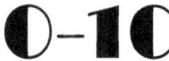 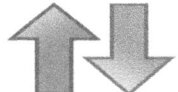

Eyebrow	So eating too much food means I want more love
Side of Eye	I don't feel very loved right now
Under the Eye	In fact, I don't feel very loveable
Nose	I just want to be loved
Chin	And if I can't feel loved, I can at least feel well fed
Collarbone	If I give up my food
Under the Arm	Then I wouldn't have food or love
Top of Head	I'm not sure I could take that.

KEEP GOING TO NEXT PAGE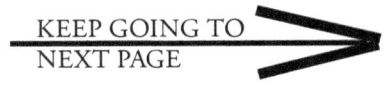

Eyebrow	Even though I have food love confusion
Side of Eye	I choose to open my awareness to feeling the love around me
Under the Eye	Even though I have food love confusion
Nose	I could choose to love myself anyway
Chin	Even though I have food love confusion
Collarbone	I am open to experiencing love in many ways
Under the Arm	Even though I have food love confusion
Top of Head	I am open to loving myself in a variety of ways, not just food

 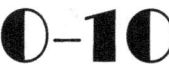 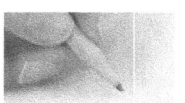

"It is during our darkest moments that we must focus to see the light." - Aristotle Onassis

I don't like to eat breakfast.

The Setup

They say that breakfast is the most important meal of the day. All of the diet books say that people who eat breakfast lose more weight than people who skip breakfast. I certainly want to lose weight more quickly and easily. I also want to be healthy. Even though I don't like to eat breakfast, I am open to honoring my body. Even though I haven't liked to eat breakfast in the past, I choose to find other foods that I might like better than what I have tried in the past. Even though I don't usually like to eat breakfast, I love and accept myself anyway.

The Tapping

Eyebrow	I don't like to eat breakfast
Side of Eye	I don't like to eat breakfast
Under the Eye	I don't like to eat breakfast
Nose	I don't like to eat breakfast
Chin	I don't like to eat breakfast
Collarbone	I don't like to eat breakfast
Under the Arm	I don't like to eat breakfast
Top of Head	I don't like to eat breakfast

 **0-10**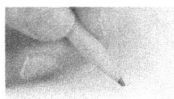

I feel unloveable.

The Setup

I don't feel like I am loveable. It isn't just because of my weight, it is because of who I am. If I am unloveable, then what is the point of losing weight? I don't think I am even loveable enough to be worth taking care of myself. It is very hard to admit that, but it seems to be a core belief. Even though I don't feel like I am loveable, I am open to learning more about where this belief came from. Even though I don't feel like I am loveable right now, and may not have been in the past either, I choose to feel hopeful that even this can change in the future. Even though I feel unloveable and think that weight loss is futile, I choose to take small steps to take care of myself until I feel more deserving.

The Tapping

Eyebrow	I feel unloveable
Side of Eye	I feel unloveable
Under the Eye	I feel unloveable
Nose	I feel unloveable
Chin	I feel unloveable
Collarbone	I feel unloveable
Under the Arm	I feel unloveable
Top of Head	I feel unloveable

KEEP GOING TO NEXT PAGE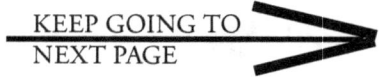

Eyebrow	I choose to examine this belief more closely
Side of Eye	Is there evidence of that?
Under the Eye	That may have been true in the past
Nose	But I doubt it
Chin	But even if it was true then, is it true now?
Collarbone	It appears that I am the one who is not loving me right now
Under the Arm	I am not taking good care of myself
Top of Head	I choose to do a better job

 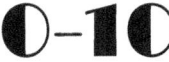 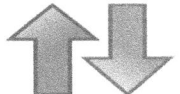

Eyebrow	There may have been a time when others didn't treat me very lovingly
Side of Eye	There may have been a time when I was unable to feel their love
Under the Eye	That doesn't really change whether I am really loveable
Nose	Those are just behaviors and feelings
Chin	My faith tells me that I must be loveable
Collarbone	It is time to claim that heritage and take better care of myself
Under the Arm	I am loveable
Top of Head	I choose to remember that I am loveable

 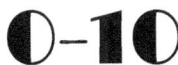 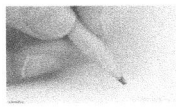

I expect weight loss to happen quickly.

The Setup

I expect weight loss to happen quickly. In fact, I expect everything to happen quickly. I am terrible at waiting. This is particularly true when it comes to weight. I certainly seem to be able to gain weight quickly. It only seems fair that weight loss should happen just as quickly. It just isn't fair. Even though I am disappointed that weight loss doesn't happen quickly, I choose to love and accept myself anyway. Even though I am disappointed that weight loss doesn't happen nearly as quickly as weight gain, I accept my thoughts, feelings, and reactions to this disappointment. Even though I expect weight loss to happen quickly, and it doesn't, I love and accept myself completely.

The Tapping

Eyebrow	I want weight loss to happen quickly
Side of Eye	And it doesn't
Under the Eye	When I am able to lose weight
Nose	It seems to happen so slowly
Chin	That I don't recognize it
Collarbone	It is easy to lose faith
Under the Arm	That it will ever come off
Top of Head	Weight loss happens too slowly

KEEP GOING TO NEXT PAGE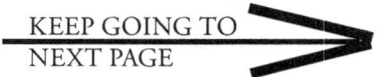

Eyebrow	I am frustrated
Side of Eye	By how slowly this is going
Under the Eye	Even though I am frustrated by my slow weight loss
Nose	I choose to remain focused on the successes I'm having
Chin	Even though I am frustrated by my slow weight loss
Collarbone	I choose to get out of my own way and allow this to happen more effortlessly
Under the Arm	Even though I am frustrated by how slow this weight loss seems
Top of Head	I choose to love myself and I accept all of my feelings about this process

   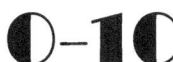   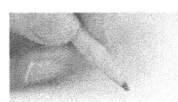

Tapping Exercise:

Begin tapping. Say these phrases aloud. Repeat each one at every tapping point before moving on.

I choose to love and accept my feelings

I look forward to a future where I can accept myself

I choose to take care of myself

I choose to remain in control of my appetite and my food

I choose to address the real life issues

I am open to clarity

I have everything I really need

I choose to accept myself

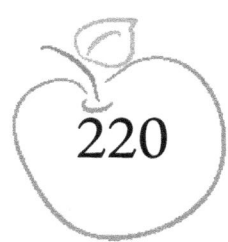

My inner child is hungry.

The Setup

I just realized that sometimes when I eat, it's not about how I'm feeling now. What I'm really doing is trying to feed my inner child, and she's hungry. I don't know any other way to feed her or soothe her. My adult brain knows that I'm hurting my adult body, but my inner child needs me and I'm trying to nurture her, even at the expense of myself. Even though my inner child is hungry, I am open to clarity about this issue. Even though my inner child is in need of love and care, I choose to find ways of caring for her that aren't destructive to my health. Even though my inner child is hungry, I deeply and completely love and accept myself.

The Tapping

Eyebrow	My inner child is hungry
Side of Eye	My inner child is hungry
Under the Eye	My inner child is hungry
Nose	My inner child is hungry
Chin	My inner child is hungry
Collarbone	My inner child is hungry
Under the Arm	My inner child is hungry
Top of Head	My inner child is hungry

KEEP GOING TO NEXT PAGE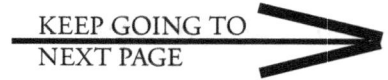

Eyebrow	My inner child is a part of me
Side of Eye	That means I must be hungry
Under the Eye	But not necessarily hungry for food
Nose	My inner child can't really be wanting food
Chin	She wants love
Collarbone	She wants comfort
Under the Arm	I want love
Top of Head	I want comfort

 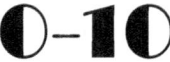 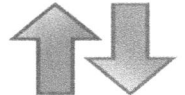

Eyebrow	I can take care of my inner child
Side of Eye	By taking care of my current self
Under the Eye	I can take care of my inner child by loving myself
Nose	My inner child deserves love
Chin	I have always deserved love
Collarbone	My inner child deserves comfort
Under the Arm	I have always deserved comfort
Top of Head	I am choosing to take care of both of us now

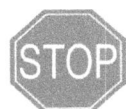 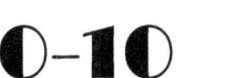 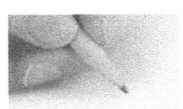

221

I know I shouldn't eat before bed.

The Setup

I know I shouldn't eat before bed. Eating late makes me gain weight. That is really true if I eat a whole meal. I got home late and I was hungry. Tired and hungry is always a bad thing for me. I wish I had been able to just have a light snack. I feel bad about having eaten too much and too late. In spite of these feelings and behaviors I love and repect myself.

The Tapping

Eyebow	I ate too late at night
Side of Eye	I also ate too much
Under the Eye	I feel bad about myself
Nose	This isn't good for my weight loss program
Chin	My self esteem has taken a hit too
Collarbone	I don't seem to have any real self control
Under the Arm	Dinner late at night is just a bad idea
Top of Head	I ate too much before bed

KEEP GOING TO NEXT PAGE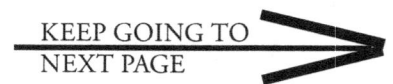

Eyebrow	I'm hungry sometimes at night
Side of Eye	I choose to forgive myself for my lack of self control
Under the Eye	I ate too much last night
Nose	And I choose to forgive myself for my lack of self control
Chin	My late night eating wasn't the best thing for me
Collarbone	And I choose to forgive myself for my lack of self control
Under the Arm	I ate too much before going to bed
Top of Head	And I choose to forgive myself for my lack of self control

   **0-10**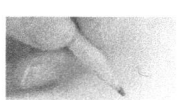

"I hated every minute of training, but I said, 'Don't quit. Suffer now and live the rest of your life as a champion." - Muhammad Ali

Food equals love.

The Setup

To me, food equals love. To give up food would mean that I'm giving up love. I don't think I can do that. I don't want to do that. Even though food equals love for me, I completely love and accept myself. Even though I yearn for food whenever I'm in need of more love, I accept myself. Even though I use food as a substitute for my need for love, I deeply and completely accept myself.

The Tapping

Eyebrow	Food equals love
Side of Eye	When I want love
Under the Eye	And I don't feel I can get it
Nose	I turn to food
Chin	When I don't feel loved or loveable
Collarbone	I turn to food
Under the Arm	For me food equals love
Top of Head	If I can't have love, I at least want to have food

KEEP GOING TO NEXT PAGE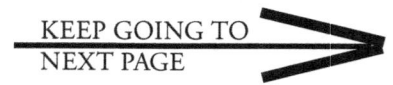

Eyebrow	Food equals love
Side of Eye	Love equals food
Under the Eye	If I can't have one
Nose	At least I can have the other
Chin	This association isn't working very well for me
Collarbone	When I'm feeling unloved and turn to food
Under the Arm	It isn't very good for my body
Top of Head	I choose to love and accept myself anyway

 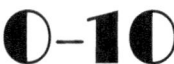 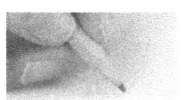

"Health is the greatest gift, contentment the greatest wealth, faithfulness the best relationship." - Buddha

I'm not an active person.

The Setup

I am not an active person. Exercise is not for me. I don't like to sweat. I don't like to breathe heavily. I don't like sore muscles. I just don't like exercise. Even though I don't see myself as an active person, I love and accept myself anyway. Even though I don't see myself as an active person, I choose to consider all of my options to improve my general health and wellness. Even though I don't see myself as an active person, and that gets in the way of my weight loss, I love and accept myself completely.

The Tapping

Eyebrow	I am not an active person
Side of Eye	I don't like exercise
Under the Eye	I don't see myself as an active person
Nose	Being active is pretty uncomfortable for me
Chin	I'm not very good at it
Collarbone	And I'm not sure I even want to be active
Under the Arm	I am not an active person
Top of Arm	I'm not sure what kind of person I really am

KEEP GOING TO NEXT PAGE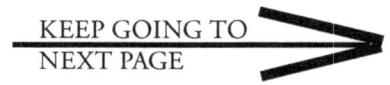

Eyebrow	I still don't think I'm an active person
Side of Eye	I never have been
Under the Eye	I probably never will be
Nose	But that doesn't mean that I can't do a few more things to get moving
Chin	I know it will be worth it
Collarbone	I want to be healthy
Under the Arm	I want to be stronger
Top of Head	I am willing to consider some new possibilities

 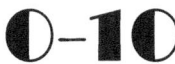 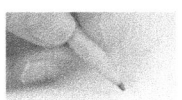

"Don't let the fear of striking out hold you back." - Babe Ruth

It's the weekend. I deserve a treat.

The Setup

Even though I believe I deserve a treat because it is a weekend, I deeply and completely love and accept myself. Even though I believe I deserve a treat since I've had a rough week, I love and accept myself anyway. Even though I want a treat and think I deserve one since it is a weekend, I love and accept myself completely.

The Tapping

Eyebrow	It is the weekend and I deserve a treat
Side of Eye	I really want a treat
Under the Eye	I believe everyone should have treats on weekends
Nose	And that includes me
Chin	I deserve a treat
Collarbone	It is the weekend and I deserve a treat
Under the Arm	I want a treat
Top of Head	And I want one now

   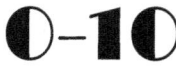   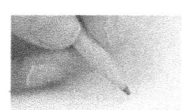

225

I feel guilty because I haven't worked out in days.

The Setup

I haven't worked out in several days. I don't feel very good about that. I believe that I should work out more often but I just don't do it. That makes me feel pretty guilty. Feeling guilty causes me to eat more. It doesn't seem to be working very well to get me moving. Even though I have all of this guilt, I deeply and completely love and accept myself.

The Tapping

Eyebrow	Guilty because I haven't worked out
Side of Eye	All of this guilt
Under the Eye	I haven't worked out in days
Nose	And I feel guilty
Chin	I feel so guilty
Collarbone	And the guilt is causing even more problems
Under the Arm	This guilt
Top of Head	This lack of exercise guilt

 **0-10**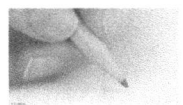

I'm searching for food nirvana.

The Setup

I'm pretty frustrated with my life. There just doesn't seem to be enough happiness. In reality, there just doesn't seem to be enough of anything. I want to feel better. I want to feel happy. I want to feel contentment. I'm seeking nirvana. Food may the only way to reach it. Even though I'm trying to reach a state of nirvana through excessive eating, I love and accept myself. Even though I'm trying to reach a state of nirvana through unhealthy eating, I choose to remain open to finding other ways.

The Tapping

Eyebrow	I'm searching
Side of Eye	I want to feel better
Under the Eye	I want to find nirvana
Nose	Food gets me close
Chin	But not close enough
Collarbone	When I eat enough to feel good
Under the Arm	I feel bad soon after
Top of Head	I just want to feel better

KEEP GOING TO
NEXT PAGE
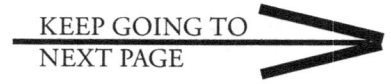

Eyebrow	I want to be happy
Side of Eye	I want to feel contentment
Under the Eye	I want to feel better
Nose	I don't know how to get there
Chin	I'm doing the best I can
Collarbone	And that doesn't seem to be good enough
Under the Arm	Excessive eating isn't really working for me
Top of Head	Eating unhealthy food isn't working for me either

 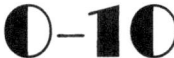 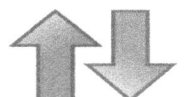

Eyebrow	Even though I've been seeking a new mood state through food
Side of Eye	I choose to remain open to other ways of finding happiness
Under the Eye	Even though I have been unhappy
Nose	I choose to allow happiness into my life
Chin	Even though I have been seeking food nirvana
Collarbone	I choose to allow contentment into my life
Under the Arm	Even though I have been searching for something to make me feel better
Top of Head	I choose to allow nirvana to enter freely into my life

 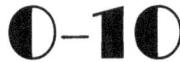 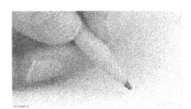

I want Girl Scout cookies.

The Setup

I went to the grocery today and there were Girl Scouts sitting at the entrance selling their cookies. I love Girl Scout cookies. I dread this time of year. The craving is so intense. Even though I am craving Girl Scout cookies right now, I choose to love and respect my health more. Even though I am craving Girl Scout cookies, I acknowledge my thoughts and feelings about this. Even though I am craving Girl Scout cookies, I choose to allow this craving to pass without acting upon it.

The Tapping

Eyebrow	This craving for Girl Scout cookies
Side of Eye	This craving for Girl Scout cookies
Under the Eye	This craving for Girl Scout cookies
Nose	This craving for Girl Scout cookies
Chin	This craving for Girl Scout cookies
Collarbone	This craving for Girl Scout cookies
Under the Arm	This craving for Girl Scout cookies
Top of Head	This craving for Girl Scout cookies

KEEP GOING TO NEXT PAGE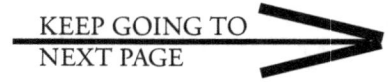

Eyebrow	I have a strong craving for Girl Scout cookies
Side of Eye	They seem to be everywhere
Under the Eye	I have fond memories of selling them when I was little
Nose	I have even better memories of eating them
Chin	Lots of them
Collarbone	I'm having an intense craving for Girl Scout cookies
Under the Arm	This strong craving
Top of Head	A craving for Girl Scout cookies

 **0-10**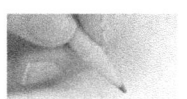

"The most authentic thing about us is our capacity to create, to overcome, to endure, to transform, to love and to be greater than our suffering." - Ben Okri

228

I'm too old to work out.

The Setup

I'm too old to work out. Exercise is for young people. Even though I really know this isn't true, and I know some very active older people, there does seem to be some programming that is holding me back. It spite of these thoughts, I love myself. In spite of these feelings, I accept myself. Even though I have these thoughts and feelings, I choose to overcome my old programming.

The Tapping

Eyebrow	I'm too old to work out
Side of Eye	I'm too old to work out
Under the Eye	I'm too old to work out
Nose	I'm too old to work out
Chin	I'm too old to work out
Collarbone	I'm too old to work out
Under the Arm	I'm too old to work out
Top of Head	I'm too old to work out

KEEP GOING TO
NEXT PAGE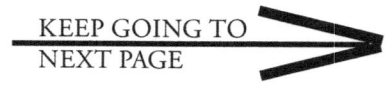

Eyebrow	I have old programming that is holding me back
Side of Eye	My beliefs may be outdated
Under the Eye	I am open to new ways of thinking
Nose	I am open to new ways of feeling
Chin	I am open to updated programming
Collarbone	I would like to enjoy exercise more
Under the Arm	I would like to allow more health and wellness into my life
Top of Head	I would like to let my body tell me what it needs

 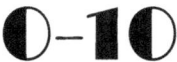 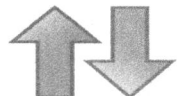

Eyebrow	Exercise helps me to feel younger
Side of Eye	Exercise helps me to look younger
Under the Eye	Exercise helps me to feel healthier
Nose	My body knows what it needs
Chin	I'm not too old
Collarbone	I'm just stuck
Under the Arm	I am opn to clarity
Top of Head	I am open to wellness

 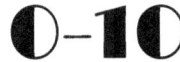 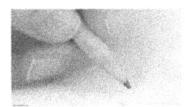

I am afraid to feel hungry.

The Setup

I'm not sure why, but I am really afraid of feeling hungry. I don't have memories of starving or ever really being without food, but the fear of being hungry is pretty intense. Even though I have this fear that I don't really understand, I deeply and completely love and accept myself. Even though I have this intense fear of feeling hungry, I accept my feelings as being legitimate. Even though I have this intense fear that I don't understand, I choose to love and accept myself and I am open to more clarity about this puzzling situation.

The Tapping

Eyebrow	I am afraid to feel hungry
Side of Eye	I am afraid to feel hungry
Under the Eye	I am afraid to feel hungry
Nose	I am afraid to feel hungry
Chin	I am afraid to feel hungry
Collarbone	I am afraid to feel hungry
Under the Arm	I am afraid to feel hungry
Top of Head	I am afraid to feel hungry

KEEP GOING TO NEXT PAGE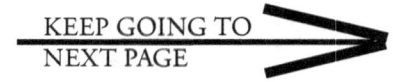

Eyebrow	I still have some of the fear about hunger
Side of Eye	I don't know where it comes from
Under the Eye	It doesn't make sense to me
Nose	I am afraid to feel hungry
Chin	Afraid to feel hunger
Collarbone	I still have some fear of hunger
Under the Arm	I would like it to go away
Top of Head	For now, I would settle for just understanding it

 **0-10**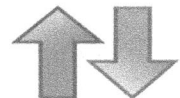

Eyebrow	I believe that if I could understand it, I could deal with it better
Side of Eye	I acknowledge that I am afraid to feel hungry
Under the Eye	I also accept that having the feeling is legitimate
Nose	Even if I don't yet understand it
Chin	I choose to treat my fear with respect and love
Collarbone	I have some remaining fear of feeling hungry
Under the Arm	And that is okay
Top of Head	I am okay

 **0-10**

References

Carrington, P. (2001) *How to create positive choices in energy psychology: choices training manual*. Kengall Park, NJ: Pace Educational Systems.

Gallo, F. & Vincenzi H. (2000). *Energy Tapping*. Okland, CA: New Harbinger Publications.

Kowalick, J. (1998). *Psychological inertia*. Retrieved July 08 2012 from http://www.triz-journal/archives/1998/08/c/

Resources

www.drleannamanuel.com

www.thetappingsolution.com

www.thrivingnow.com

About The Author

Dr. Manuel is a clinical psychologist working at Kirtland Air Force Base in Albuquerque, New Mexico. Previously she was in private practice in Beavercreek Ohio where her clients were diverse and spanned all ages. Always looking for ways to move people to higher levels of functioning in life, Dr. Manuel has combined traditional psychological practice with ancient martial arts, energy work, and activity-based therapies.

Dr. Manuel is a woman who is actively looking for opportunities to expand her boundaries and enjoy life. Her formal training is as a registered nurse and clinical psychologist. She is also a Reiki master, martial artist, and Meridian Tapping practitioner.

On the homefront, Dr. Manuel is the mother of two handsome, talented, and loving sons that are now exploring the world on their own terms. Those sons have doubled the size of her family by adding beautiful and intelligent women to their lives. She is also the mother of a beautiful daughter who has lived with her heavenly family since infancy.

She has a mission. That mission is to recognize and develop the unique brilliance in every individual with which she has contact. And that includes you. It is her hope that you will find some morsel, no matter how large or small, that will move you toward a deeper and more satisfying connection with yourself and the Universe. Dr. Manuel is continually challenging herself to become the very best that she can be. That is her challenge also to you. We all have the tools at our disposal. Now all we have to do is use them. Just keep tapping.

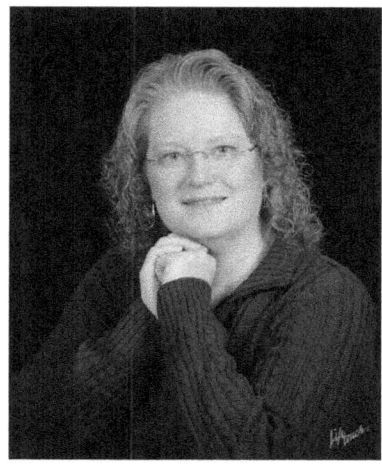

www.ingramcontent.com/pod-product-compliance
Lightning Source LLC
Chambersburg PA
CBHW080241290526
45790CB00005B/1663